"Self-care is a survival skill that's re
world. *The Yoga Almanac* turns the p
that links us to the cycles of nature, weaving in the astrological calendar
and fostering a connection to source energy. A gorgeous guide for recon-
necting to the rhythms within ourselves and all around us."

—**Ophira and Tali Edut (The AstroTwins)**, founders
of www.astrostyle.com

"An indispensable compendium of practical philosophy, thought-provok-
ing rituals, and functional anatomy, *The Yoga Almanac* is a one-of-a-kind
seasonal guide to developing a practice of clarity, presence, and alignment
with integrity. Whether you're a student, teacher, or curious about what
yoga and meditation might do for you, *The Yoga Almanac* is a key resource
for us all."

—**Elena Brower**, best-selling author of *Practice You*

"As a voracious reader and longtime practitioner, I've read a whole lot of
books about the practice of yoga. But I've never come across a book so
unique in perspective combining the philosophy of yoga and of astrology.
I was instantly inspired to dive deep into this book and it's now a resource,
and muse I'll always be returning to. I highly recommend this book to
reinvigorate both your yoga practice and daily life."

—**Mary Beth LaRue**, cofounder of Rock Your Bliss,
and international yoga instructor

"A contemporary, real-life, accessible, educational, all-inclusive master-piece, *The Yoga Almanac* has become my go-to manual for creative inspira-tion, and a steady guide for staying focused on my personal spiritual journey. A timeless treasure that belongs on the bookshelves of students and seekers everywhere."

—**Robert Sturman**, artist and photographer

"We do yoga because we long to truly know and care for ourselves in a more loving way. But how can we do that in the middle of our crazy, busy lives? Lisette Cheresson and Andrea Rice show us how in *The Yoga Almanac*. They offer ritual, poses, stories, and weekly practices designed to wake us up, help us navigate the world with kindness and grace, and bring us home to our inner wisdom. Reading this book is like going on a self-care retreat, guided by two wise and loving teachers."

—**Linda Sparrowe**, former editor of *Yoga Journal* and
Yoga International; and award-winning author of six
books on yoga, including *Yoga At Home*

"*The Yoga Almanac* is a creative perspective that provides a foundation for practitioners who are interested in understanding the ways in which our relationship to understanding astrology inform the relationship we culti-vate with the physical body. This is a great resource for anyone looking for a fresh, innovative, and meaningful way to move deeper into a yoga practice."

—**Chelsea Jackson Roberts, PhD, E-RYT**, cofounder
of Red Clay Yoga

THE YOGA ALMANAC

52 Practices *and* Rituals *to* Stay Grounded Through *the* Astrological Seasons

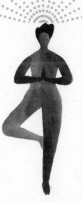

LISETTE CHERESSON | ANDREA RICE

REVEAL PRESS

AN IMPRINT OF NEW HARBINGER PUBLICATIONS

Publisher's Note

This publication is designed to provide accurate and authoritative information in regard to the subject matter covered. It is sold with the understanding that the publisher is not engaged in rendering psychological, financial, legal, or other professional services. If expert assistance or counseling is needed, the services of a competent professional should be sought.

Distributed in Canada by Raincoast Books

Copyright © 2020 by Lisette Cheresson and Andrea Rice

       Reveal Press

       An imprint of New Harbinger Publications, Inc.

       5674 Shattuck Avenue

       Oakland, CA 94609

       www.newharbinger.com

Cover design by Sara Christian; Cover background photo by Andy Holmes on Unsplash; Cover geometric abstract shape by Freepik.com; Interior Illustrations by Ryan LeMere; Acquired by Ryan Buresh; Copy edited by Marisa Solis

The "Astrological Wheel of Life" is copyright Andrea Rice. Design by Mollie Earls.

Translation of "Salutation to the Dawn" by Kalidasa by W. S. Merwin, currently collected in SANSKRIT LOVE POEMS. Copyright © 1977 by W. S. Merwin, used by permission of The Wylie Agency LLC.

Lines from *The Upanishads* (translated by Eknath Easwaran, founder of the Blue Mountain Center of Meditation, copyright 1987, 2007) are reprinted by permission of Nilgiri Press, P. O. Box 256, Tomales, CA 94971; http://www.bmcm.org.

Library of Congress Cataloging-in-Publication Data on file

Printed in the United States of America

22   21   20

10   9   8   7   6   5   4   3   2   1   First Printing

This book is dedicated to all the seekers on the journey of self-realization; to the students devoted to this lifelong practice and the teachers who help to guide us there.

Contents

SUMMER:
A Time to Flourish and Thrive
Cancer   Leo   Virgo

AUTUMN
Embracing Transition and Finding Equilibrium
Libra Scorpio Sagittarius

WINTER
The Quiet Inward Journey
Capricorn   Aquarius   Pisces

Introduction

Human beings are governed, in ways subtle and obvious, by rhythms of the natural world. We rise with the sun and rest with the moon. We honor our familial and ancestral heritages with cultural occasions throughout the calendar year. Many of our emotional impulses are a response to the ebb and flow of the seasons—whether we're conscious of it or not.

Spring is apt for renewal, for planting seeds of intention that take root in the soil of our personal inner gardens. Summer calls for cultivation, as those seeds begin to blossom, to celebrate the fruits of our labor with levity and play. In autumn, we begin to let things fall away as we harvest what was sown, share in abundance, and express gratitude. The quiet solitude of winter draws us inward to reflect, reintegrate, return, and release.

Becoming aware of seasonal cadence brings us closer to the natural world. By reintegrating with these rhythms, we deepen our shared connection and strengthen our bonds. Most important, we reconnect to primal wisdom and glean higher, spiritual insight. Through practice and ritual, we begin to harness this alchemical potential.

Whether you're new to yoga and meditation, a long-time practitioner, or an experienced teacher, *The Yoga Almanac* is a vehicle to navigate these continuing cycles of change. With weekly rituals, exercises, poses, and journaling prompts, all readers—new to yoga or not—may consider this book a cursory crash course in how to apply yogic wisdom and theory to daily, modern life.

For the yogi-curious, *The Yoga Almanac* serves as a comprehensive entry point to develop a self-study practice that will help you stay balanced as the world turns. For the seasoned practitioner, it is a foundation for furthering your knowledge of philosophy and spiritual sciences by viewing the effects of nature's rhythms through a yogic lens. For the teacher, the fifty-two weekly explorations will serve as thematic fodder for your classes and writings, which—as has already been tested by us, your authors—will resonate on a universal level with your students.

The popularity of yoga asana—or physical yoga—has exploded in recent years. But contrary to what many nonpractitioners may think, yoga asana is not an exercise fad geared toward a specific demographic or physicality. Yoga is for everyone, and any *body* can do yoga. Many people shy away from a yoga practice, believing that they're not flexible or strong enough, because of what they see in mainstream advertising and on social media. If you ask just about anyone what yoga is, you would likely hear a slew of answers—many of which are far from the truth.

Put simply, yoga is the practice of knowing yourself and understanding your real nature through taking wise and skillful action in the present moment. It is learning—or relearning—how to *be here now.* "Yoga" means union. It begins on a mat or seated on a cushion in meditation. In time and with practice, we learn how to incorporate this mind-body-spirit connection into our daily lives. Physical yoga is only one of eight "limbs" of the practice. You are a yogi when you consider your relationship to yourself and the world around you—not necessarily when you perform superhuman feats of strength or flexibility.

This book is in no way a complete glossary of yoga philosophy or terminology. Vedic philosophy relies heavily on oral tradition—even in modernity—and much of what we've curated in *The Yoga Almanac* is up for modern interpretation. For example, Patanjali's *Yoga Sutras* (circa 100–300 CE), is generally considered the basis of yogic theory, though there is no definitive translation. The same goes for Hindu mythology. While some religious texts are referenced, this book is not meant to serve as a resource for dogma but rather as a tool for personal enrichment. Neither of the authors grew up in a Hindu household, and, like our interpretation of the *Yoga Sutras,* this book represents decades of yoga study and practice, our combined knowledge of the spiritual sciences, and, as journalists, some good old-fashioned research. The information we're offering here is a jumping-off point for your own self-study, which—whether you're just beginning or continuing—is a lifelong journey of learning and discovery.

The physical poses we offer are a suggestion to embody the seasonal and cosmic themes we've presented for a given week. Our intention is to provide the most accessible postures we can, since we believe that "advanced" asana is often rooted in the ego rather than spirit. We've also included namesake legends based on Hindu mythology, as well as translations of Sanskrit where applicable. Physical explanations are intended for readers with a basic comprehension of functional anatomy, as well as for new practitioners who would like to begin a safe, sustainable practice with a foundational physical understanding.

Yoga is a wonderful way to get back in touch with your body and discover how it can function optimally: what types of movement patterns might serve, and which ones could cause harm and should be avoided. When we connect with our physicality, we're more readily able to grasp the inner workings of our minds and spirits. That's when the *yoga* actually starts to happen.

We choose to work with the Western tropical zodiac wheel—which was philosophized by the Ancient Greek astronomer Ptolemy—to give more context to the physical postures and themes we propose. Ptolemy put forth geocentric theory: that Earth was the center of the universe. We don't purport that astrology has hard scientific merit, but we agree with Ptolemy's idea that the colossal celestial bodies in our solar system could have an energetic effect on human behavior and temperament down here on Earth. This is why we've deemed the incorporation of astrological themes in *The Yoga Almanac* as "cosmic embodiment": our method for embodying the energy of the heavens above into our bodies and minds.

There are three astrological sub-seasons within each of the four seasons that make up the twelve signs of the zodiac wheel. During each astrological season, when the sun is in a specific sign (as viewed from our vantage point here on Earth), we experience the energy of that corresponding sign. For example, the first day of spring coincides with the beginning of Aries season; Aries is the first sign, and is metaphorically much like spring.

The Western tropical zodiac does not offer much discussion of planetary rulers for chakras, the seven subtle energy centers of the body that run along the spinal cord. The existence of chakras was first theorized in the Vedas, ancient classical Indian text, as cakras, or "wheels" of light. During our research, we learned that the ancient system of Vedic sidereal astrology—incorporated before the outer planets (Uranus, Neptune, Pluto) were discovered—did in fact associate planets with chakras. We've noted this relationship where applicable, as well as the parts of the body associated with each sign of the zodiac.

To further invoke the celestial qualities of astrological archetypes, we've also assigned each chapter a weekly ritual as a means of
taking the themes off of the mat. As the very first sutra asserts, "Yoga
is happening now." It's not a practice that happens in a vacuum or
solely in a studio but rather when you take it out into the world and
into your daily life. Some of the rituals may become part of your
weekly, monthly, or even annual routines. Some may not resonate,
and that's okay too. The practice here is to discover what works for
you and what doesn't—and to feel free to get creative and develop
your own personal practices accordingly.

Closing each chapter is a short poem in the form of a dharma
talk, indicated by an om symbol (ॐ). This sacred Sanskrit hiero-
glyph depicts the primordial sound of the universe; the essence of
everything. Om is often chanted at the beginning or end of a class. A
dharma talk comes from the Buddhism lineage, however, in which it
is customary for teachers to offer lectures or very short sermons to
students to open or close a meditation practice. Yogis may recognize
the tradition from a modern yoga class when teachers read a short
passage, typically during Savasana (the final resting pose that culminates a physical practice) or during an opening meditation. Teachers
reading this book may choose to use the dharma talks in their classes;
others may simply find these few stanzas helpful as a short and sweet
chapter summary to help digest the information.

You may choose to use *The Yoga Almanac* in a number of ways,
whether in seasonal succession from start to finish, or beginning with
whatever time of year you happen to pick it up. You may, however,
choose chapters at random depending on your mood or present circumstance. Just as the world turns from the birth of spring into the
lushness of summer, the shedding of autumn to the death of winter,

so too can this book be used cyclically again and again. Just as we typically begin practice as a child and close as a corpse, a reintegration into natural rhythms reflects the cycle of birth, death, and rebirth, known in Sanskrit as samsara.

Each time we come to the mat—and take those lessons into the world—we're moving forward, spinning along the wheel of life, participating in our own cycles of change and growth. We hope this book generates personal inquiry and, ultimately, helps guide you toward a deeper level of self-realization and understanding.

In light,

Lisette & Andrea

SPRING

Revival, Renewal, and Growth

Aries • **Taurus** • **Gemini**

"Look to this day,
For it is life,
The very life of life.
In its brief course lie all the truths
And realities of your existence;
The bliss of growth
The glory of action, and
The splendor of beauty;
For yesterday is but a dream
And tomorrow is only a vision."

—Kālidāsa, Salutation to the Dawn

Though spring encompasses the beginning of the astrological calendar—and serves as the starting point for this book—this season is a transitional one. It's a phase of renewal, apt for planting the seeds of intention from the start of a new calendar year that we wish to nurture and watch blossom. As tree branches return to life and buds burst forth, the soil thaws and fields are sown. The lively energy of spring inspires us to seek new beginnings, launch new endeavors, and lay the foundation for what we seek or desire to cultivate in our lives. We find ourselves pulled to clear out the clutter and fling open windows. As the days become longer and, in the Northern Hemisphere, the Earth's axis turns closer toward the sun, we integrate the introspective wisdom of winter's contemplation. Spring marries that darkness with rays of light that illuminate the very landscape of the soul.

The vernal equinox, on March 20 or 21 each year, corresponds with the start of Aries season. As the first sign of the zodiac symbolized by the Ram, Aries is considered the astrological baby and is synonymous with fresh starts. Aries is ruled by the celestial warrior Mars (one of two love planets). The action-oriented energy of this phase rekindles any forward-moving momentum that may have stalled since the start of the new year.

Ayurveda, yoga's sister science, categorizes the year into three seasons, rather than the four of the Gregorian calendar, each of which corresponds to the most prevalent dosha. An Ayurvedic dosha can be thought of as a pervasive energy in the body that manifests as physical temperament. The three doshas are kapha (earth), pitta (fire), and vata (air). Ayurveda posits that a person may be more apt to act a certain way given the prevalence of one dosha over another. These are not fixed qualities—a person may be more heavily kapha one season and pitta the next.

Spring straddles the end of airy vata season, characterized as dry and cool, and the earthy, wet, rooting qualities associated with the kapha dosha. Kaphic energy is dense and grounded, sensual and steady, akin to traits of Taurus season, which begins April 20 or 21 and is represented by the patient Bull. Once we have harnessed the frenetic and fertile energy of the start of spring, we can settle into stability, as our roots are planted firmly in fecund ground. Taurus is ruled by Venus, the love planet associated with sensibility and practical luxury.

Beginning around May 21, Gemini season winds down the frenzy of spring and is characterized by relationships and community. The sign of the Twins is chatty by nature and ruled by the communication planet, Mercury. This last stage of the vernal cycle prepares us for the abundance of the coming months, teaching us to enjoy working with others as we look toward the levity and playfulness of summer.

Coming off the heavy heels of Piscean energy, Aries season tends to be more singularly focused on personal ambition and drive, whereas Gemini season is lighthearted and gregarious. Being aware of these fluctuations in the external world engenders a better understanding of our emotional states and any psychological or physiological transformations we may experience.

In the Native American Medicine Wheel tradition, spring is the season of the East, associated with the rising sun and the potential for possibility as we embrace the unknown. It is a time of curiosity— some animals emerge from hibernation, others hatch and emerge into the world. Spring is a season for considering our own metaphorical rebirth, as we shed our winter layers and find equilibrium between the shadows of colder months behind us and the blazing spirit of what is yet to come.

BIRTH

Mastering Unconscious Inheritances

As sentient beings with a prefrontal cortex, the gift of human life comes with a great paradox: we are born with the blessing of infinite potential and the curse of primal ignorance. We unconsciously default to our primary nature of karmic inheritance: the unique patterning we bring into this world. How we're conditioned by society throughout our upbringing reinforces these patterns, for better or worse. We can choose a lifetime of unconscious repetition, or practice the process of illumination by acknowledging our patterns and eventually breaking free. Each time we do, we experience a metaphorical death and are born again.

These psychic "scars" are known in Hindu philosophy by their Sanskrit name, samskaras, and hinder our capacity to know ourselves. They are the heavy burdens we carry, the negative inner critic that holds us back, the unhealthy behaviors we repeat. Ignorance is false bliss; it is separate from the pure bliss awareness of knowing ourselves. It is easier to stay in the dark—where it is comfortable, safe, and easy—than it is to navigate the emotional and psychological challenges of stepping fully into the light. We must traverse the shadows and witness what has been previously hidden from view. We may not always like what we see.

Patanjali's *Yoga Sutras* describe the five kleshas as the collective obstacles that keep us from understanding our real nature. The first, avidya (ignorance), is described as one's inability to discern between permanence and impermanence, pure and impure, bliss and suffering, the true self and the non-self. Avidya sets the stage for the four hindrances that follow: asmita (egoism), raga (attachments), dvesha (aversions), and abhinivesha (fear of death). Through practice, we reestablish a lifeline back to the true self and may spend a lifetime working through the other obstacles.

For many yoga and meditation practitioners, the first opportunity to break through the barrier of ignorance may occur on the mat or cushion. Through the practice of presence, we witness our own prana, qi, or life force pulsating within. In sutra 1.1, Patanjali directs that yoga is happening *now;* it is a birth into the present moment as the inherited, false parts of ourselves unravel and fall away.

On March 20 or 21 in the Northern Hemisphere, the vernal equinox coincides with the start of Aries season and marks the reset of the astrological calendar—a metaphor for new beginnings and a cosmic rebirth. Aries is the "baby" of the zodiac and can be childish at times. Yet, this youthful mentality reminds us of the power of potentiality. Ruled by Mars, the impassioned love planet, Aries is symbolized by the initiative-driven Ram and is associated with the head.

PRACTICE

Child's Pose
(Balasana)

Child's Pose is symbolic for entering into the world in a vulnerable position. When we begin practice in this shape of being born, we nurture our connection to source. It is a pose we revisit throughout practice, a shape in which we feel at home in our bodies.

Child's Pose may be practiced with knees together or wide, arms released by your sides. This relieves tension in the upper body to invite natural flexion in your thoracic spine. To support your knees and hips, place a blanket between your seat and the backs of your knees. Extended Child's Pose is practiced with arms reaching overhead, facilitating shoulder extension. You can also stack your palms beneath your forehead, with your elbows out to the side, to support your head and neck.

Child's Pose grounds us into our root (muladhara) chakra and activates the third-eye (ajna) chakra by pressing forehead to the ground.

THIS WEEK: WHAT ARE YOU INVITING IN?

Spring is an opportunity for renewal and rebirth—for planting seeds to nurture and for witnessing the unending cycle of growth and change. It is also a reminder that we cannot be born again until we experience a death—a shedding of old layers, habits, and outmoded beliefs. Springtime is ripe for new possibility.

Make a list of all that you're ready to bring into your life, along with what must be released in order to make space for these opportunities. Then organize them into Yes or No columns. The Yes column includes everything that you're saying a resounding yes to—what you want more of in your life. The No column includes everything that needs to be released so that each item on your Yes list may be made manifest. An ideal time for this exercise is on or near a new moon, which heralds the beginning of a new lunar cycle.

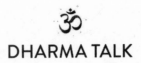

DHARMA TALK

Wherever you are now,
whatever you are feeling
or thinking,
it will eventually change
and transmute.
For each and every
waking moment
is a chance to be
born anew.

AWAKENING

Planting Seeds in Fertile Ground

Spring is an apt metaphor to plant seeds for the blossoming of an idea. Days become longer, animals awaken from hibernation, and fields that have lain fallow since harvest are given new life. More than just a new beginning, the season asks us where we intend to focus as we awaken to the possibilities before us.

In Hinduism, Shakti is the primordial energy of the universe. This is associated with the divine feminine and the goddess Shakti, or Devi, Lord Shiva's omnipotent consort, but it is not specific to gender. When we realize that everything is made of Shakti, we can more readily awaken to an embodied state of experiential bliss.

Yoga is a practice of awakening this energy, depicted as a coiled snake at our root (muladhara) chakra at the base of the spine that travels up the shushumna (central spinal column), toward our crown (sahasrara) chakra. Patanjali's eight limbs are directives to live a life in pursuit of this awakening as we continue along the cycle of birth, death, and rebirth (samsara)—until we reach reunification with the divine.

Practice asks us to examine the internal blockages that keep us from knowing ourselves. This requires not only determination but joyful willingness. By accepting our physical limitations and celebrating our personal progress, we become active participants in our lives. Anchored in this foundation, we plant potent seeds from which satisfaction and freedom from our own inhibitions may grow. Just as the root systems of plants and forests are interconnected, so too are we. Yogic theory posits that there is no freedom from suffering—no awakening to ultimate truth—unless all beings are free.

Awakening belongs to the domain of Aries. Ruled by Mars, Aries energy compels us to initiate the changes we want to see. Aries is a fire sign—its motivation needs to be both fueled and contained in order to regenerate. Symbolized by the Ram, Aries pushes hard and fast, rather than taking a measured approach. Beware of burnout—give the seeds you plant ample time to take root.

PRACTICE

Forward Fold
(Uttanasana)

Translated from Sanskrit, "ut" means "intense"; "tan" is "to stretch or lengthen." Logical Aries rules the brain, face, and head. A gentle inversion, Forward Fold places the head below the heart, increasing blood flow to the face. Forward Fold stretches the fascia, the connective tissue that encapsulates muscle and bone, of the back body. The plantar fascia of the feet is also manipulated as the soles anchor into the ground.

   Included in both Sun Salutations A and B, Forward Fold is ubiquitous throughout a typical vinyasa class. It's worth noting that practicing Forward Fold doesn't mean you have to touch your toes or the floor, or keep your legs perfectly straight. Maintain a soft—or significant—bend in the knees to stabilize and strengthen your hamstrings, which in turn supports a healthy and functional lower back and neutral spine. Your feet can be together or hips-width-distance apart, depending on your bodily structure. Arms can hang heavy or reach for opposite elbows.

Hinging at the hips engages the sacral (svadhisthana) chakra, our center of passion and sexuality. Stabilizing the spine by engaging abdominal muscles activates the solar plexus (manipura) chakra, the fiery center of Aries's proactive vitality and the seat of digestive organs. Forward Folds are said to improve digestion and relieve menstrual cramps.

THIS WEEK: BREATH OF FIRE PRANAYAMA

We awaken when we clear the cobwebs of metaphorical sleep from our minds. Breath of Fire, or kapalabhati ("skull shining breath"), calms the nervous system and expands lung capacity. It is an energizing pranayama and a foundational practice in Kundalini yoga.

Come to a comfortable seat, and place the hands on the abdomen. Inhale deeply, and begin short and quick evenly cadenced exhales and inhales (two to three per second), placing emphasis on the exhale. The belly button will pump as the diaphragm moves. Keep breathing like this for twenty to thirty seconds, and then deeply exhale. Repeat as is comfortable.

Note: this is an advanced pranayama. If you're new to the practice, twenty to thirty seconds may be ambitious. Pause or slow your rhythm of breath as needed.

DHARMA TALK

We sleep to wake,
night falls for dawn.
In the darkness,
she coils and quiets,
prepares to awaken
with first morning light.
As she rises and sings her
siren song, so too do rise
other snakes in the field.
Stretching toward the sun,
they reach and grow as one.

SPONTANEITY

Freedom from Inhibition

Life is a balance between meticulous planning and letting the magic unfold. Nature is spontaneous, as are all creatures, including humankind. The demands and desires of modern society have infringed upon our innate curiosity by overplanning and overscheduling in pursuit of success, fortune, and fame. Reclaiming this curiosity awakens the potential for infinite possibility.

To be spontaneous is to live freely without self-imposed constraint or social inhibition. It is to ebb and flow and be open to what is possible, rather than avoid or resist certain situations that deviate from our normal routines or make us uncomfortable. Spontaneity is different from acting on impulse, which is often volatile and driven by impatience. To be spontaneous is to be responsive—to surrender to the undercurrents of the universe and ride the waves that come our way. Spontaneity is a state of natural flow.

Chinese philosophy describes Tao as the driving life force behind creation and existence. Known as "the way," Tao is the essence of spontaneity and governs the principles of yin and yang. To unite with the spontaneity of Tao is to practice noninterference, to allow life to unfold without manipulation. Laozi—the great Chinese philosopher and author of the Tao Te Ching—said that all beings ought to develop and change in accordance with noninterference by following their own nature, which is brimming with Tao (Laozi 2004). Regardless, Laozi also acknowledges humanity's underlying resistance to spontaneity.

Hindu philosophy discusses the concept of brahmacharya, the behavior or ideal use of one's energy that is in alignment with Brahma, the god who created the world and all living beings. Brahmacharya explains that asserting control over our impulse toward excess can lead us to wisdom and vitality. It takes courage to overcome our inherent desires to be more, want more, and have more, and willpower to let go of our need for perfection. Presence gleaned on the mat or cushion teaches us to surrender to all that is, assuring us that our lives are unfolding as they should. We need not always know where we're going, yet we can acknowledge where we've been and where we are now.

Spontaneity is a combustible trait of Aries, an impassioned—and sometimes impatient—fire sign ruled by the warrior planet Mars and symbolized by the courageous Ram. A motivated and a leadership-oriented cardinal sign, Aries will sometimes force its way through obstacles. Aries rules the head and is ambitious, aggressive, a bit playful, and eccentric—fearlessly blazing its own trail.

PRACTICE

Arrow Lunge
(Anjaneyasana Variation)

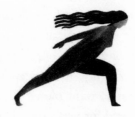

This adapted version of a Crescent Lunge (see page 93) activates the muscles of the back body (posterior chain). The dynamic shape can be explored either with the back knee lowered or lifted, with the arms overhead or stretched behind, or with palms interlaced. Arrow Lunge strengthens the glutes, hamstrings, lats, shoulder girdle, and lower back. You can explore movement from a Crescent Lunge to Arrow Lunge with your arms overhead and back knee down, and then lift your back knee, hinge forward, and reach your arms back by your sides.

As you focus your "aim" by extending through your head, you retain a strong and neutral spine, and facilitate an opening of the crown (sahasrara) chakra. Consider what it is you're powerfully aiming toward. Embody the qualities of the unstoppable Ram in bold pursuit of your dreams.

THIS WEEK: SPONTANEOUSLY IMPROVISE

As John Lennon crooned, life happens while you're making other plans. Sometimes you've got to let go of plans and go with the flow.

Choose a night on the calendar and make a plan with a friend to be spontaneous. You can cover the bases, such as time and meeting place, but keep things loose from there. Whether it's dinnertime or you're meeting for a cocktail or tea, drive or walk to a neighborhood with some different options.

The key here is not to think it, but to *feel* it. Try to release yourself from any expectation of how the night is going to go—be open to the idea that where you land may not necessarily be what you had in mind. Exploring unfamiliar territory teaches us to accept the discomfort of the unknown. When the activity is over, consider keeping the night going and make another spontaneous decision about where to go next. Allow the events to unfold organically as you relax into flow.

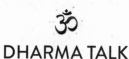

DHARMA TALK

There is underlying order
despite random acts
of cosmic chaos.
To give into flow
without thinking but feeling,
we accept our place amid the chaos.
From the well of spontaneity
springs divine synchronicity.
And the internal compass points
toward infinite possibility.

4

LEADERSHIP

Living in Dharma to Guide Others

Leadership is the ability to motivate a group of people to work toward a common goal. Leaders are remembered for what they build and create—and how successful they are at uniting the collective imagination. They have a clear sense of purpose and direction, and they adhere to certain principles as a road map to get there. Leadership is not limited to people who command—and desire—attention, however. We are each in command of our own life.

The Vedas describe dharma as a way of living in accordance with sadharana dharma, a universal ethical code, and svadharma, an individual one. The practice of yoga awakens our personal dharma—purpose in this life—and thus our potential. Living in sadharana dharma accepts the interconnectedness of experience. To accept svadharma is to follow our personal moral path.

Practice challenges us to seek realization and self-knowing, and to approach the journey with humility. When we reach a point of stagnancy or our bodies change, practice asks us to innovate. Humility, perseverance, innovation, and compassion are all characteristics of a respected leader. Life, however, is more complicated than that. At times, leadership requires certain sacrifices for the greater good. In the Bhagavad Gita, Krishna explains to Arjuna that he must fight in a battle against his family because his svadharma in that moment was as a warrior. To live in the dharma of a noble president, for example, a leader may need to risk their popularity for the benefit of their country.

Leadership belongs to Aries, the cardinal sign that leads the astrological year. Aries energy is enterprising, marking an ideal moment for embarking on a new journey or taking more initiative at work or with a project. Ruled by Mars, the planet of war, Aries's leadership can border on aggression if not tempered with empathy. The grit and determination that keeps Aries marching into battle are traits that many leaders possess.

PRACTICE

Chair Pose
(Utkatasana)

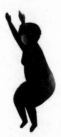

Utkatasana comes from the Sanskrit word "utkata," meaning "fiercely proud or difficult." Its English name is for its shape, sitting into an invisible chair. The chair, or throne, is a significant symbol in Hindu mythology, as it was customary for civilians to sit on the floor. In the Ramayana, Rama's stepmother forces his exile for fourteen years so that her son Bharta could ascend the throne. Knowing that it was not his dharma to be king, Bharta placed Rama's sandals in the empty seat to hold the rightful leader's place until he could return.

Chair Pose can be practiced with your feet hips-width apart, your big toes touching, or any other stance that feels natural and stable. The posture improves shoulder flexibility and mobility. Maintain a neutral spine as you reach your arms wide and overhead to either frame your ears or your face. Engage your glutes and hamstrings to activate your transverse abdominis (deep core) muscles to sustain this deceptively difficult posture.

Chair Pose fires up the solar plexus (manipura) chakra, center of purpose and identity. As you sit back into your imaginary chair, take the seat of your personal power and call upon the blazing energy of Aries.

THIS WEEK: CONSIDER MENTORSHIP

There is truth in the axiom that in order to truly learn something a person must be able to teach it. Leadership, at its core, is the ability to empower others, to build and to create. In a mentorship relationship, these lessons go both ways.

Research a local branch of a national organization, such as Big Brothers Big Sisters of America or MENTOR. If something like this isn't available, contact your local library or school and offer to volunteer with after-school or tutoring programs.

What are you learning from the mentees? How have you noticed your perceptions and expectations evolving? How does mentoring others help you self-actualize your potential for leadership?

DHARMA TALK

To lead is not to force others to follow
but to realize that
your fullest potential
has always been within.
To lead is to walk strong in dharma,
to know where you are and where
you'd like to go,
trusting not just plans
but process.
We are all born leaders.
To lead is to learn
how to become.

GROUNDING

Steadfastness Through Any Storm

Contentment is inner peace that comes with the cultivation of acceptance. Recognizing the impermanence of any situation, good or bad, relieves us from the fear of an unknown future, from any guilt or shame of the past. Yoga is a practice of fortifying the neural and physiological patterns of equanimity that ground us into the present moment. We learn to become comfortable and strong in our place in the world—temporary and fleeting as it may be.

In sutra 1.12, Patanjali introduces two key teachings to maintain this composure: abhyasa, persistent practice, and vairagya, non-attachment. We must put forth the effort but be unattached to outcome. We do this by learning to be in the here and now. Persistent practice creates steadfastness—the courage to keep going, keep trying, even against all odds.

On the mat, we come home to our bodies through breath, establishing patterns of serenity and composure. From this foundation, we may begin to explore the process of self-actualization through the practice of non-attachment, which leads us toward contentment and acceptance.

Tibetan monks and nuns practice the sacred art of the sand mandala—an artistic masterpiece made from individual grains of colored sand—as tangible representation of this concept: no matter how many days it takes to create the masterpiece, it will be wiped clean.

In his 1943 paper, "A Theory of Human Motivation," psychologist Abraham Maslow introduced the human hierarchy of needs. The theory posits that when basic needs are met (water, food, shelter), we are able to move on to psychological needs (relationships, professional accomplishment) and then fulfillment needs (creative and abstract pursuit). When we are grounded physiologically and emotionally, we set the foundation for personal development.

Grounding is a theme for stable and rooted Taurus. Reliable and dependable, this fixed sign brings steadiness and resolute persistence to any project. Taurus is symbolized by the Bull, a sacred animal in several mythologies, representing patience and fecundity. As the second sign in the zodiac, Taurus is the first feminine sign, evoking energies of security and tradition.

PRACTICE

Tree Pose
(Vrksasana)

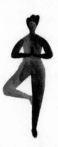

Tree Pose is a physical metaphor for rooting to rise. The Buddha sat patiently beneath the Bodhi tree to achieve enlightenment. In a Hindu myth, Bhagiratha stood on one foot for a thousand years to persuade the gods to allow the goddess Ganga to descend and release the souls of his ancestors. His steadfastness brought the River Ganges to Earth, her waters with powers to break the cycle of reincarnation.

Balancing is a practice, and it may take some time exploring the edges of your feet—shifting the weight from ball mounds to heels—before you gain a sense of your foundation. Bring the sole of your foot above or below your knee, and engage your gluteal muscles to enhance your stability and activate your transverse abdominal muscles (the ones you feel when you cough). Maintain neutrality in your hips as you lift your hands to your heart or extend your arms overhead like branches.

Tree Pose activates the foundational seat of the root (muladhara) chakra. A balanced root chakra is the base for a life of equanimity and contentment. Opening the hip rouses the sacral (svadhisthana) chakra, our center of relationships. Tree Pose also awakens the solar plexus (manipura) chakra, our self-confidence and stability. Allow yourself to wobble; give yourself permission to fall. Just as storms test the resolve of our steadfastness, balancing poses teach us to give in to the nature of flux.

THIS WEEK: CRAFT A FAMILY HISTORY

Families form from all corners of relationships. Consider a group of people with whom you share a narrative—who, collectively, have played an important role in who you are. They could be blood related, friends, members of a book club, coworkers, et cetera. Choose a way to tell your story—an audio library or a digital album of videos, perhaps—and interview each person about what that specific time in your life meant to them. Share the project with your "family."

If you're fortunate enough to have them with you, you could alternatively gather everyone together to share stories in person. In this case, you could create a scrapbook of the event to memorialize your history. Pay close attention to each person's story—are you surprised by what they remember?

ॐ

DHARMA TALK

We are as strong as the roots
that anchor us to personal soil.
Foundations are the fonts
from which our truest selves spring.
Equanimity enables us to find
calm in any storm, love in any loss,
to find promise of dawn
even in a starless night.

TRUST

Confidence in Times of Uncertainty

Risk yields boundless possibility, yet transition challenges our sense of security and self-worth. We procrastinate with excuses: we'll move forward when debts are paid off, when we've practiced enough, when we've obtained the certificate. To trust is to take a leap of faith—to hurdle over the misplaced belief that once everything is in order, risk taking will become less scary. Whether it's a new job, a move to a new place, becoming a parent, or pursuing a dream, when has anyone ever been truly "ready"?

Trusting in the process is to honor intuition. In a yoga practice, we tap into the wisdom of our bodies. Meditation teaches us to breathe through the mind's chatter and settle into the serenity of stillness. This increases our capacity to stay calm and at ease, even in the face of uncertainty or fear.

In sutra 1.17 Patanjali describes the stages that lead us to samadhi, or reunification with the divine: vitarka (reasoning), vicara (reflecting), ananda (rejoicing), and asmita (understanding the true self). Practice is a vehicle that guides us toward samadhi, providing glimpses of our true nature, and is not a process that can be rushed. In sutra 2.19, Patanjali explains the four levels of natural matter, from what is seen to what is unseen. Though we cannot see the scent of a flower, we trust in our sense of smell.

What we chase after in modern life—fortune, position, beauty—is fleeting. Focusing our efforts on obtaining what is impermanent results in dissatisfaction, shackling us to the material world. When we understand the world's suffering as temporary, we trust in the unfolding of existence and live from a place of embodied peace.

The theme of trust arrives just after the frenetic awakening of Aries season and grounds us into the stabilizing energy of Taurus. An earth sign, Taurus is symbolized by the steady but stubborn Bull that knows when to maintain pace and when to charge. Themes of resistance may surface during this phase. Drawing on the patient energy of Taurus, we relearn to trust life. But it doesn't happen overnight; committing to trust is a lifelong daily habit.

The Yoga Almanac

PRACTICE

Cobra Pose
(Bhujangasana)

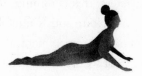

Cobra Pose is an ideal substitute for Upward-Facing Dog (see page 103) and can be practiced high or low to the ground, depending on spinal and shoulder mobility or arm strength. In a modification commonly cued as Baby Cobra, less emphasis is placed on spinal extension and drawing the elbows toward straight. Try not to drop your head back, which compresses your cervical spine.

If you have wrist issues, it's not necessary to press your palms into the floor. Instead, breathe into your back and front body. As your belly fills with air, allow that buoyancy to lift your chest and forehead from the ground as you float your palms beside you, keeping your elbows bent by your sides. You can press into your pubic bone and thighs to generate spinal extension—the beginning of a backbend. If there is tension in your lower back, lower down slightly and engage your glutes to protect and strengthen that region.

Lying on the belly activates the root (muladhara) and solar plexus (manipura) chakras, centers of ancestral memory and personal power. Cobra's opening across the chest and throat also stimulates the heart (anahata) and throat (vishuddha) chakras. Taurus rules the throat and neck.

THIS WEEK: TUNE INTO YOUR GUT

Your gut is widely recognized as the second brain, and there's scientific evidence to trust your gut (Sonnenberg and Sonnenberg 2015). While it does not possess cognitive thinking abilities, your gut contains an ecosystem of bacteria that communicate with more than one hundred million neurons—your body's microbiome. The health of our gut impacts our mood or temperament; the more in tune we are with our gut, the more trust we are able to cultivate.

Tapping into gut feelings engenders confidence in difficult decisions, regardless of outcome. Focus on a decision you're facing, perhaps one that revolves around beginning something new. Tune into your body and pay attention to any sensation that arises in your belly when you consider possible outcomes. Write the feelings down—whether it's butterflies or nausea, excitement or dread, resistance or ease, and so forth. Without overthinking it, can you take some form of action to follow through? If your gut said, "Don't do it," what might you do instead?

DHARMA TALK

No doubt the universe is
unfolding as it should; no
doubt your place is secure,
your dharma deserved.
Leaps of faith are resounding
acceptance of that which
we may not understand.
To trust is to surrender to your
rightful place in the world,
same as unshakable trees
bending to shifting winds.

DEVOTION

When Loyalty Meets Accountability

Devotion is a practice of faith and loyalty. It's unwavering commitment—to an obligation, job, cause, or practice. It's to be reliable and have integrity, to accept personal responsibility and hold ourselves accountable. Devotion is a pursuit of reasonable goal setting, dropping excuses, and overcoming procrastination. When we do the work—whether for career or personal development—we fulfill our sense of purpose and duty. We honor our unique mission of becoming the person we most want to be.

Hinduism describes devotion as a path of love or bhakti, a spiritual practice dedicated to a god or guru. Hindus perform a puja, a prayer ritual as an act of worship or to honor a guest or commemorate an occasion. In Buddhism, devotional meditations are practiced to purify the mind and live in the presence of the master. The Buddha was known for discouraging excessive worship by his followers, however. Placing any spiritual leader on a pedestal can cloud judgment and disrupt the development of our unique character.

A devotional is a book or publication typically found at a church, temple, or mosque that contains a reading for the day or week to be used during prayer or meditation. The reading serves as fodder for contemplation. This very book you're reading could be considered a devotional—though its intention is to use religious references as personal enrichment only.

Other tools for a devotional practice include altars, iconography, and prayer beads. It is worth noting the appropriation of Hindu or Buddhist japamala beads as adornment in the West among yoga and spiritual communities. Traditionally, the strand of 108 mala beads is used for repetition of prayer or mantra, similar to a Catholic rosary.

Themes of loyalty and devotion are invoked during Taurus season, a romantic cycle that favors ritualizing routines. Ruled by Venus, the lavish love planet that adores decadence, Taurus has energy that is methodical yet beautifying, bringing magic to the mundane. Taurus rules the neck and physical body, and is known for taking its sweet, sensual time. Pragmatic and practical, Taurus is a grounded and sensible earth sign. When we are reliable in our personal responsibilities, Taurus reminds us that we can hold others—friends, family members, coworkers—to similar accord.

PRACTICE

Seated Neck Stretch

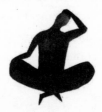

There are twenty-six muscles in the neck that attach in and around the cervical spine. The neck holds the weight of the head, about ten pounds on average. Our cervical spine tends to extend forward from its normal upright and neutral position as a byproduct of the digital evolution. The "tech neck" pandemic results from frequently looking down at handheld devices or hunching forward in front of a screen. Seated Neck Stretch helps counteract this stress and strengthen the region—and serves as a reminder to hold your head up high and be your own guru.

From a tall, comfortable, and supported seat, relax your lower back and lift from root to crown as you draw your ears back. With your chin parallel to the floor, turn your head from side to side. Then drop one ear toward your shoulder without force, and then repeat on the other side. To help relax the trapezius muscle, gently place the same-side hand on your crown and tilt your chin slightly upward. These slight rotation and flexion movements in your cervical spine can assist in unblocking your throat (vishuddha) chakra.

The Yoga Almanac

THIS WEEK: HOLD YOURSELF ACCOUNTABLE

Spring is an ideal time to take stock of the new habits we created at the start of the calendar year, noticing what we've prioritized and what we've let slip away. Is there a goal you put on the back burner that you'd like to revisit? Whether it's sticking to a meditation practice, fitting in a regular exercise routine, eating better, or saving money, can you recommit to this habit now?

Consider your goal in the devotional or ritualistic sense—as part of your regimen—because it is nourishing the person you are becoming and not just another item on your to-do list. Better yet, enlist a friend or family member to help hold you accountable with regular check-ins.

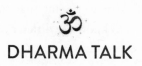

DHARMA TALK

Devotion
is love in motion,
as we tap into the ocean
beneath chaos and commotion.
Our infinite well
where energy dwells
replenishes our core,
every fiber and cell,
as devotional hearts
beat and swell.

PLEASURE

Intentional Sensuality

The pursuit of pleasure is complicated. Our bodies are hardwired to respond to the senses, as our brains flood with "happy hormones": endorphins, serotonin, dopamine, and oxytocin. Pleasure is a biological feedback loop of desire and satisfaction. Reliance on external stimulation, however, leads to longing, addiction, and regret, and blind hedonism that may cause internal and external conflict. Intentional sensuality is to know the difference between healthy and unhealthy indulgences.

In yogic theory, "ananda" is a Sanskrit word that refers to the state of pure bliss. Paramahansa Yogananda, author of the seminal *Autobiography of a Yogi* (1946), taught that ananda is an eternal pleasure. Bliss comes from a deep well of innate joy. Yoga and meditation teach us to go beyond the mind's fleeting desires and draw from that well. In so doing, we experience a shift from our default doing and thinking mode to a grounded state of feeling and being.

Yogananda's teachings echo sutra 2.7, in which Patanjali asserts that temporary sensory pleasure is the source of attachment. When we chase after impermanent things, we become dependent or attached, and we forget that the potential for contentment exists within. Sutra 2.15 continues with the pursuit of pleasure, resulting in pain if denied and fear of loss if gained.

Patanjali describes moral and ethical codes for living in the Sutras, known as the yamas and niyamas. Brahmacharya is the yama that instructs tempering sensory stimulation in favor of the more permanent pleasure of samadhi, divine connection. Though brahmacharya traditionally implies abstinence, it can be interpreted as a directive to temper the need for external gratification and relish in life's small pleasures instead. The world is bursting with opportunity to embrace beauty. Whatever brings you joy in life—music, food, social activity, sex—the trick is to not yearn for it.

Pleasure and sensuality belong to Taurus, the bodily and earthy sign of the zodiac. Symbolized by the fertile Bull, Taurus is aroused by physicality but remains rooted in stability even as senses are engaged. Ruled by Venus, planet of love and pleasure, you may find yourself particularly drawn to sensual pursuits this time of year. Striking a balance between celebrating your relationships and appreciating your material possessions, rather than clinging to them, is the challenge during this season.

PRACTICE

Happy Baby Pose
(Ananda Balasana)

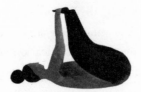

In Hindu mythology, Dasaratha was an aging king who had three wives but no heirs, so he called on the gods to help his wives conceive. Dasaratha gave Vishnu's fertility potion to his first wife, Kaushalya (whose name in Sanskrit means "well-being" or "happiness"), who shared it with the others. Kaushalya gave birth to Rama, an avatar of Vishnu. When we are unattached to our bounty and share our resources, we awaken the teacher within.

Happy Baby Pose can be practiced by grabbing for the feet, ankles, or shins, depending on your range of motion, with your knees bent and just wide of your hips. Rock gently from side to side if that helps your hip flexors relax. Happy Baby also strengthens your hamstrings and can relieve lower-back discomfort.

Opening the hips stimulates the sacral (svadhisthana) chakra. A balanced sacral chakra is necessary to enjoy the fleeting sensations of passion, sensuality, and pleasure.

THIS WEEK: SAVOR AN INDULGENCE

Regardless of temporality, the pursuit of pleasure need not be rushed. To tap into what pleasure means to you—and to develop a detached relationship to it—you must master the art of savoring. For this ritual, home in on something seemingly inconsequential that you do every day, such as drinking a morning tea or coffee.

Take a moment to engage all five senses. How does the tea smell? How does the warm cup in your hand feel? If you are using a splash of cream or almond milk, watch the way it swirls into your beverage. Breathe deeply. Sip slowly. When you take the last sip, remind yourself that the pleasure isn't just the tea but how it makes you feel in the moment. Enjoying the impermanence of the little things is good practice for creating a healthy sense of detachment.

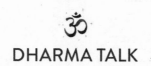

DHARMA TALK

Pleasure is not found in attainment
but in the approach.
Our senses are barometers
to shifting winds of change.
Life's joy is not in arriving but in pursuit.
When what we seek is
understood as fleeting,
fulfillment is lasting and whole.

SUSTAINABILITY

Going the Distance

The Peruvian American author Carlos Castaneda said that the amount of effort required to be miserable or strong is the same. It's the nature of the mind to fixate on problems and create issues when there are none. Self-imposed woes beget exhaustion; stress is physically and mentally draining. Yoga and meditation practices exercise and strengthen the resolve of body and mind to overcome proclivities toward negativity and stress.

To lead a life of longevity is to enhance mind-body endurance. Physical activities like yoga, brisk walking, running or jogging, dancing, swimming, cycling, playing team sports, or taking the stairs increase our physical durability. Developing endurance—particularly in today's sedentary culture—strengthens the heart and lungs, maintains healthy circulation, and decreases our risk for heart disease or stroke and even diabetes.

But a strong body can still burn out when the mind is left unchecked. Just as a muscle in the body atrophies with lack of use, so too can the mind spin out of control when not exercised. Mental-boosting activities such as meditation increase mental durability and the capacity for concentration and contentment. Developing mental stamina allows us to tackle our to-dos with less energy depletion and to maximize our output. Many elite-level athletes have adopted meditation practices that emphasize breathing techniques to make them more efficient. When we have more endurance, we can more readily deliver oxygen to the bloodstream.

Springtime is apt for mental and physical training, and the grounding energy of Taurus can help us go the distance. Symbolized by the Bull, slow and steady Taurus is patient yet persistent. As the zodiac's first earth sign and a stabilizing fixed sign, Taurus encourages us to find ease, wherever we are on the path. Taurus is governed by Venus and attunes us to our sensuality. Taurus rules the throat and neck, and is associated with physicality.

PRACTICE

Tribal Lunge

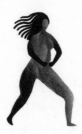

This dynamic shape comes from the Bowspring method, a practice that emphasizes the body's natural curves for optimal functional movement to facilitate forward bends, backbends, and side bends to allow maximum length and minimum compression to the spine.

Tribal Lunge is reminiscent of Warrior II (see page 65), but it maintains a bend in the back knee and does not rotate the pelvis forward. The foot placement is similar to Warrior II, but in Tribal Lunge the stance is narrower. The back foot (called Earth Foot in Bowspring) remains anchored as the front foot faces forward. The front knee is only slightly bent and angled inward in line with the toes of the back foot.

Begin standing with the knees slightly bent and draw a slight curve into your lower back to bring your spine to neutral. Step one foot back to a wide stance so that your back heel is slightly turned out, and your back knee and toes point slightly in toward your midline. Keep your ribcage vertical and both knees bent, aligning your back knee with your back toes and your front knee over your front foot.

Hands can be kept at your heart, or you may stretch arms out wide or in front of you with elbows bent and fingertips facing each other (as if you were holding a beach ball), similar to first position *en avant* in classical ballet. You can also make gentle fists. Try shifting your weight from one leg to the other, bending one knee deeply and then the other, and then switch legs by stepping forward and then stepping back with the other foot, building momentum as you go.

As you root your lower body to load the springiness of your legs, there is a sense of weightlessness and mobility in the upper body. This anchored stability can help open the root (muladhara) chakra.

THIS WEEK: SHOP SUSTAINABLY

The Dalai Lama (1990) wrote that the universal responsibility of humanity is to the longevity of our environment, the planet we call home. Leading a sustainable lifestyle is more accessible than ever. When it comes to protecting Earth's precious resources, we can all do our part as conscious consumers.

With myriad eco-friendly products and options, there are many shifts we can make to reduce our carbon footprint and minimize our environmental impact. Some ideas:

- Check product labels to ensure they meet Environmental Protection Agency and Federal Trade Commission standards (i.e., the official USDA Organic seal, the Green Seal, EcoLogo, NRDC, or Fair Trade Certified)

- Boycott products that test on animals or are harmful to ecological systems and/or wildlife

- Conserve water

- Eat less meat

- Go plastic-free

- Carpool, bike, or take public transportation

- Use wind or solar power

- Vote for representatives who lobby for change

Can you commit to living more sustainably this week? How about this month, year—or indefinitely?

DHARMA TALK

Root down to rise
and move with grace.
Responsibly take
and sustainably make
decisions that ensure
abundance for generations.
Each choice you make
has a lasting impact
on your mind and body,
on our planet and fate.

PARTNERSHIP

The Power of Conscious Connection

Whatever your beliefs or desires about marriage or monogamy, we humans appreciate meaningful relationships. Partnership is more than someone to wake up with or someone to take care of us when we're sick. A healthy partnership is a mirror for personal understanding. Strong emotional responses to a partner's behavior may reveal deep, unacknowledged truths about ourselves.

In the West the word "tantra" conjures sexual hedonism or sex without release; in India, tantra is sometimes associated with black magic. Tantra is actually the canon of texts that describe yogic and meditative practices resulting in spiritual liberation. Tantric rituals are sensual exercises—such as prolonged touching or listening—to consciously connect to our partner and become fully absorbed in the present. These practices generate deeper intimacy and build emotional intelligence.

The goal of tantra is to unify Shakti (feminine) energy with Shiva (masculine) energy. Some interpretations of tantra suggest that orgasms are an expulsion of divine energy and thus should be avoided. Between 200 to 400 CE, most likely in Northern India, Vātsyāyana wrote the *Kamasutra,* the world's oldest extant book on eroticism.

More than simply a manual of sexual positions, the *Kamasutra* is a treatise on the art of living, with instruction on relationships, partnership, and enjoyment of our sensual bodies.

Tantric sex and the *Kamasutra* are often confused. Tantric rituals employ sensuality as a means to enlightenment; the *Kamasutra* asserts that sex can be pure pleasure. The *Kamasutra* calls for equal participation, emphasizes the power of touch and foreplay, and encourages intimate playfulness. All of these help create a foundation for a partnership that gives us glimpses of our truest natures.

Partnership falls under Gemini's domain. Symbolized by the Twins, Gemini energy is playful and adventurous, teaching us to seek synchronicity and collaboration. Ruled by Mercury, the planet of communication, this air sign emphasizes the power of openness—particularly with significant people in our lives. Gemini is known for sexual creativity and embracing sexual exploration. We may find ourselves craving deep and fulfilling relationships during this time of year, perhaps a kindred spirit, whether intimate or platonic. Gemini rules the shoulders and upper arms—in order to be able to hold someone else, we must first know how to truly hold ourselves.

The Yoga Almanac

PRACTICE

Supported Shoulder Stand
(Salamba Sarvangasana)

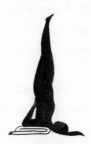

Supported Shoulder Stand can reap the same benefits as any inversion when practiced against a wall. This shape helps to circulate lymph fluid, bolstering the immune system.

Place a blanket about a foot from the wall. Walk your feet up the wall and begin to gently roll onto your shoulder girdle, the foundation for this pose. Press into your triceps and bring your hands to your lower back for support as you tilt your pelvis to lift your hips. Extend your legs, as your shoulders can readily support them. You can also practice the shape from a supported Bridge Pose by placing a block underneath the back of your pelvis, and then lifting your feet to extend your legs upward.

Shoulder Stand stimulates the throat (vishuddha) chakra, the seat of expression. An open throat chakra ensures that we are able to communicate what we desire—with our partner or otherwise. The throat is the energetic bridge of our heart, the center of love and relationships, and our upper chakras, the seats of intuition and divine union.

THIS WEEK: THE ART OF MIRRORING

To practice radical compassion with a partner or loved one, we must not only listen and hear but empathize. Choose a kindred spirit in your life who you trust and whose relationship with you has been tested. Face each other, and recall a moment in your shared history—maybe a blissful memory, perhaps an argument. One person speaks first and explains their memory of that moment, uninterrupted. Rather than simply repeating what was said, the second person pauses, ruminates, and then reflects back to the first person with a summary of what they shared. Repeat the exercise by taking turns.

Interpreting memories in this way not only teaches us where we can continue to improve as one half of a relationship but reveals insight into how the other person feels and thinks.

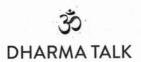

DHARMA TALK

We are interconnected creatures,
symbiotic as the forest to rain.
Partnership teaches us not only
who we are but how to be, how to
live, and how to love.
Seeking the vulnerability of intimacy
teaches us how to be strong.
Nurturing relationships with others
is the nature of our innermost self.

ADAPTABILITY

Our Mutable Natures

Despite tendencies to resist the unknown, humans are changeable beings. Our kaleidoscopic natures adapt to fluctuating circumstances, yet the overthinking mind, a side effect of advanced cognitive abilities, can sabotage this primal process. Biological adaptations are behavioral or physiological byproducts of genetic mutation and evolution. It is not the most intellectual of species that survives, nor is it the strongest. Rather, it is those most adept at adapting to an ever-changing world.

The nature of yoga is adaptation. Patanjali's *Yoga Sutras*—the foundation for yogic theory—was adapted from an oral lineage in Sanskrit; physical asana has also been adapted. "Vinyasa," for example, gets its name from the Sanskrit terminology "nyasa" ("to place") and "vi" ("in a special way"). This notion of divine arrangement was adapted as the model for Pattabhi Jois's six-series Ashtanga Vinyasa Yoga method in the mid-twentieth century. Jois's physically demanding, athletic style made its way to the West in the 1980s, where it was adapted as a form of aerobic exercise. The nonalignment system of ashtanga became problematic for many Western practitioners—particularly the forceful hands-on assists. Alignment-based vinyasa yoga was born—the wildly popular style common today.

Unfortunately, this adaptation has had negative effects as well. Universal alignment cues have become watered down like a game of telephone. Rather than building the structure for a pose first, some vinyasa teachers attempt to put students into a shape and then reverse-engineer biomechanics to "fix it." Further, and particularly with the rise of social media, mainstream vinyasa is popularized by teachers who prioritize creative flair and notoriety over safe functionality. The proliferation of images that show hypermobile contortionists in inaccessible shapes draw thousands of likes—and dollars. Imitation of these images has created an epidemic of yoga-related injuries. This is a false representation of what yoga really is. And it alienates people who, based on what they've seen on social media, believe they're not strong or flexible enough, or don't have the "right" body type to practice.

On the flip side, yoga has been adapted for marginalized populations. Practitioners have developed specialized practices for disabled persons, trauma survivors, veterans, and cancer patients, among others. There's also been a rise in teachers who are returning to the essence of yoga with the intent to make the practice more accessible and universal through skillful action, discernment, acceptance, contentment, and present-moment awareness. Because yoga truly is for every *body*, it is our responsibility as yogis to continue to adapt our practices accordingly.

Adaptability falls in the domain of curious Gemini, who bores easily and is known for changing its mutable mind. Symbolized by the Twins, Gemini is ruled by Mercury and governs communication. Gemini is associated with the hands, fingers, arms, lungs, and nervous system. There is never a dull moment during Gemini season, as synergy sparks among like-minded people and we're encouraged to adapt to new surroundings.

PRACTICE

Modified Four-Limbed Staff Pose
(Chaturanga Dandasana)

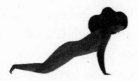

The hypnotic element of a vinyasa class often leads to escapism. The predictability of common cues (such as, "Take a vinyasa") causes more tuning out than in, as we fall into familiar habits and patterning. Modified Four-Limbed Staff Pose—commonly referred to by its shortened Sanskrit name, Chaturanga—is especially precarious, because it's an anticipated transition that links sequences together. When a student has not developed sufficient upper-body strength, they might either support their torso with their elbows beneath their ribcage, or collapse into a banana back, compromising the safety of their lumbar.

To adapt Chaturanga, lower your knees and place your palms just wide of your elbows, maintaining a neutral spine. Begin by lowering a third of the way down without collapsing your chest or shoulders. Press back up, then lower again, maybe halfway down. Either press back up and transition back to Downward-Facing Dog (see page 214), or shift forward to lower all the way to the ground. From here, Baby Cobra Pose (see page 34) is an option to facilitate a gentle opening of the chest to activate the heart (anahata) chakra, or you can opt out and press into your palms and knees to return to your starting position.

THIS WEEK: CHANGE YOUR MINDSET

When we cling to comfort and familiarity, we stall personal and professional progress, and cease to develop our character or sharpen our skills. Examine a current source of stress in your life, maybe a rut you feel stuck in. Changing a situation begins with an adjustment in attitude; a small internal shift spurs external transformation.

Write down any negative self-talk associated with the problem you're examining. Change this language by making statements instead of complaints. Can you develop a new dialogue surrounding your situation that supports the change you wish to see?

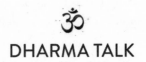

DHARMA TALK

We adapt when we know
when to go with the flow
or swim against the stream
and smash the status quo.

CONNECTIVITY

Our Vast Neural Network

Interconnectedness exists all around us and in us. Our brains contain roughly one hundred billion neurons (or nerve cells), each connected to ten thousand other neurons that generate up to one thousand trillion synaptic connections to transmit information. The interconnectivity of neurotransmission brings to mind what Friedrich Nietzsche may have meant when he said, "Invisible threads are the strongest ties."

Your brain is like a muscle—it needs exercise. With practice, yoga trains the brain to more readily defer to the parasympathetic nervous system through concentration and movement. This rewiring increases neuroplasticity, the ability of the brain to generate—or sculpt—new neural pathways and repair damaged ones.

Neuroplasticity has been witnessed in rehabilitation programs for patients with traumatic brain injury or paralysis. The Canadian psychologist and "father of neuropsychology" Donald Hebb proposed that repetition forms and reinforces neural pathways attributed to learning and memory. His work has been paraphrased by the clever rhyme: "What fires together, wires together" (Keysers and Gazzola 2014).

Our habits, thoughts, and behavioral patterns strengthen neural networks, whether positive or negative. If you're stressed out about a particular situation, your brain will fortify neural networks that reaffirm that stress. Spending time in quiet, contemplative inquiry can illuminate any deep-seated inherited patterning. In psychology, this patterning is known as the default mode network. Your default mode can be a place of imagination and introspection, but if you've experienced trauma, it can also be an uncomfortable, dark, even self-destructive state.

Meditation trains your brain to set a new default mode, increasing the gray matter density in the brain, which is responsible for memory, empathy, and stress. Contentment and happiness are learned skills that meditation and yoga help us hone. The practice of presence and acceptance reestablishes our sense of connectedness and belonging.

Connectivity is Gemini's wheelhouse, the sign of the chatty Twins and the quick-witted master of interpersonal connection. Ruled by Mercury, the messenger planet governing communication, Gemini is driven by partnership, reminding us that how we show up for others begins with how we show up for ourselves. Known for being a bit mentally preoccupied at times, Gemini rules the nervous system and is also associated with the hands.

PRACTICE

Wide-Legged Forward Fold
(Prasarita Padottanasana)

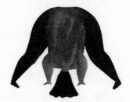

Forward Folds activate the rest-and-digest function of the nervous system. As the mind enters a relaxed state, we experience relief from anxiety and stress. Wide-Legged Forward Fold strengthens the hamstrings, calves, and ankles, as the lower back releases and hips open. There are many ways to explore this shape to stretch the shoulders and upper back, and strengthen the wrists. You may interlace hands behind your sacrum and stretch overhead, clasp hands behind your skull, or place palms to the ground and reach for opposite feet or ankles.

Rooting the hands and feet into the earth sends the sensation of prana or qi throughout the circuitry of your body like an electrical current. By softening your knees as you hinge forward, a gentle rush of blood flows to your head and relieves tension in your neck and shoulders, creating a chain reaction to open the throat (vishuddha), third-eye (ajna), and crown (sahasrara) chakras. The groundedness of the shape can also balance the root (muladhara) chakra.

THIS WEEK: MUSIC AS MEDITATION

Einstein once said that had he not been a physicist he would have been a musician, for he often thought in music. Studies in biomusicology (Clayton, Sager, and Will 2004) and brainwave entrainment have shown that music can help heal the psyche. We are hardwired to respond to music.

Entrainment induces a relaxed state with enhanced focus, similar to meditation, by using a pulsing light or sound, which aligns the brainwaves with a certain frequency. Power down your devices and put on a favorite playlist. Pay attention to the beat. Sit or lie on the floor, stretch, keep your eyes open or closed, and let your mind wander. Notice your body's natural responses and impulses: the tap of a foot, a bob of the head, the urge to dance. Freewrite about how you feel afterward.

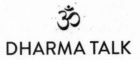

DHARMA TALK

Dispatches from a beating heart are
messages that pulse through veins.
Neurons fire missives like
wisdom in an oak tree extending from its trunk,
capillaries of swaying branches.
Great webs of life are electrified
with streams of consciousness,
the microcosm of the macrocosm
consciously communicating
in divine connection.

13

COMMUNITY

Our Bridge to the Self

The desire for and importance of social interaction is written in our DNA. The animal kingdom is flush with species that create complex communities. Elephants live in organized herds and participate in rituals like funeral rites; whales share songs from one pod to the next. Humans are no exception.

Our definition of community, however, is shifting. We self-organize based on background, belief systems, and socioeconomics rather than on location—as was the case before the Internet. While there are obvious social pitfalls to stratified organization (the echo-chamber effect of social media, for instance), the building of community is not just a biological imperative but a spiritual one.

Buddhists believe and give allegiance to the Buddha, dharma (his teachings), and sangha (the community of believers), traditionally considered as a monastic order. Vietnamese monk and renowned peace activist Thich Nhat Hanh (2008) wrote that sangha is the most important of these—and not limited to monks and nuns. A person's sangha, he wrote, is made up of their family and friends, hopefully people who help them on the spiritual path. A person is the seed. Their sangha is the soil.

We become the people with whom we surround ourselves. Just as a partner can be a mirror to your truest self, so too does community shape both worldview and action. A personal sangha should be a reflection of one's values and beliefs, and share in the pursuit of any personal goals. If we are surrounded by people who hinder our personal development, we may find ourselves stunted.

Psychoanalysts would call communities that are dissonant with personal pursuits or goals ego-dystonic. Ego-syntonic situations or communities are those that support a worldview compatible with your view of the self and your personal values. A necessary component of an intentional life is an ego-syntonic community, a sangha, that encourages and fosters individual growth.

Community falls under the realm of Gemini, the social butterfly of the zodiac that thrives on interpersonal relationships. A mutable sign, Gemini believes that there is room enough for all of us. This, of course, is a great inclusionary quality but one to be wary of when considering the idea of sangha. Gemini energy may be accepting of ego-dystonic relationships that can hinder one's journey rather than support it.

PRACTICE

Warrior II (Virabhadrasana II)

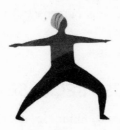

Warrior poses are named for the evolution of the thousand-eyed, thousand-limbed monster Virabhadra, formed from a tuft of Shiva's hair. Daksha, a powerful priest, held a yagna (a ritual sacrifice) and did not invite his daughter Sati or her husband, Shiva. Angry with her father, Sati threw herself into a fire in retaliation. Shiva was so devastated that he ripped a tuft of hair from his head, from which sprang the thousand-headed warrior Virabhadra, who decapitated Daksha with his mighty sword. Despite his being the supreme deity, Shiva's exclusion from the event created a monster. Even deities need community.

Warrior II is a foundational pose, often used as a transition in vinyasa classes. Keep a shortened stance to protect your sacroiliac (SI) joints, which connect your hips to your spine, and ground into the outer edge of your back heel while keeping a slight bend in your back knee to prevent hyperextension. It is not necessary to square your hips. As your chest opens, your gaze (drishti) can focus just past your front extended arm—but only if this does not cause strain in your neck. This pose strengthens leg muscles and stretches the groins.

Warrior II activates the sacral (svadhisthana) chakra. The seat of relationships, an open sacral chakra is essential for the development of meaningful connection. The slight stretch across the chest engages the heart (anahata) chakra, allowing you to plug into an ego-syntonic community that supports your personal truths.

THIS WEEK: A JUST-BECAUSE CELEBRATION

We often turn to our communities—family, friends, teachers, studios—when in the face of challenge. When things are easy, we sometimes take our communities for granted. To foster feelings of goodwill and support for the bad times, it's important to cultivate relationships with our communities during the good.

Think of an activity you enjoy doing—going out to eat, savoring a warm cup of tea or glass of wine, venturing out to a specific museum or park—something you may normally reserve for a special occasion. Invite someone to be your guest for the afternoon. Make it a point to express your gratitude for their presence in your life. When you part ways, encourage them to do the same for someone else.

DHARMA TALK

Coming together in sangha
grounds us into our strength.
Fostering appreciation for
those who help us grow
encourages us to reach new heights.
Holding community close is
what allows us to feel held.
Supported as we are in this space,
we are able to then support others.

SUMMER

A Time to Flourish and Thrive

Cancer ◉ Leo ◉ Virgo

"A harvest of peace is produced
by a seed of contentment."

—Proverb

Summertime inspires passion, prosperity, and play. The levity of the season is reflected in longer days, shorter nights, and warmer weather that encourages us to get outside and explore the beauty of the natural world. We bask in the light of what makes us happy: that which ignites our inner fires and feeds our souls. Trees and vegetation settle into their lushest green, flora blossoms into deep and vibrant hues, and fauna teems with life. Fields become flush as crops ripen for peak season harvest, and a sense of richness and opportunity abounds.

In this season of bounty, our practices become a conduit for exploration of the abundance within; a means to tend our inner gardens so that we may maximize the intake of our spiritual harvest. As we cycle through anticipation of summer getaways and embrace lazier days, we will inevitably find ourselves alongside the back-to-school frenzy as the season begins to wind down.

In the Northern Hemisphere, the summer solstice, also known as midsummer, occurs on June 20 or 21, when the Earth's north pole tilts on its gravitational axis toward the Sun at 23.5 degrees. This, of course, gives way to the longest day of the year—a moment marked by ritual and celebration throughout history. Ancient civilizations from Egypt and Rome to Stonehenge and Machu Picchu commemorated the solstice for its significance in agricultural pursuit as well as spiritual exploration.

The solstice encourages us to look within, to cultivate and support inner radiance by turning to rituals and practices that nurture personal growth and receptivity to the world around us. It is a time to invite fire back into our lives and an opportunity to burn away all that we have outgrown. We are, after all, children of the sun. Much like the brightest star in our solar system, we too create life with our own light.

In 2015, the United Nations officially recognized the first International Day of Yoga, an annual celebration held, not so coincidentally, on the summer solstice. The commemorated day acknowledges yoga as a bridge across cultural divides and reminds us that the yoking of body and mind, when applied to the global body politic, can be a way to heal our psychic wounds on a universal level.

The summer solstice also marks the first day of Cancer season in astrology. As the fourth sign of the zodiac wheel, Cancer symbolizes the divine feminine and is ruled by the moon. It is associated with the third-eye (ajna) chakra in Vedic astrology. During Cancer season, taking time for introspection and nurturing the self can help us get back in touch with our heart's true desires. At the solstice, we can recognize the sun as well as the moon and reflect on the balance of male and female in our lives and in the world around us.

The third-eye chakra is governed by the moon and the sun: the feminine and masculine principles. Leo is ruled by the sun, and its fiery, masculine forces are also associated with the third eye. Leo season begins on July 22 or 23 and encourages us to express our most heartfelt passions with fierce, unabashed confidence. This dramatic, heart-opening phase is also associated with the heart chakra.

Virgo season begins at the height of summer, typically on August 21 or 22. Virgo is synonymous with cleanliness and detoxification, and is symbolized by the Virgin or Maiden carrying a shaft of wheat. Ruled by Mercury, the planet of communication, Virgo is synonymous with the throat (vishuddha) chakra. Virgo is associated with the digestive organs, signifying a cycle to purge and purify in anticipation for the coming fall season.

Ayurveda describes summer as having an excessive pitta quality in the atmosphere, which can shorten fuses and lead to frustration and angry outbursts. (Pitta season runs from approximately July through October.) It is why "cooling" practices are so often prescribed during this phase, because as Earth heats up, so do our minds and bodies.

In some medicine wheel traditions, summer is associated with the South. Animals of the South, the eagle and the wolf, share summer's valuable lessons of strength and resolve, of bravery and fulfillment. Summer encourages us to look within, to reignite our passions and align with a sense of higher purpose. It is the season for bold pursuit of our greatest truths, so that we may step into our fullest power and potential.

14

SELF-CARE

Finding a Home in Yourself

Bubble baths and dark chocolate may be antidotes to a hectic world—but self-care is more than indulgence. It's about slowing down and tuning into the subtle wisdom of your body and your mind. It's coming home to yourself, relishing in the hallways of your imagination, rejuvenating without external stimuli, and trusting that doing so is not selfish.

The summer solstice is an apt time to welcome ourselves home to the practices that nurture our bodies and nourish our souls. Through the ritual of showing up to these practices, whatever those may be, we remain anchored to the core of our being as we navigate the peaks and valleys of life.

Practicing self-care creates bodily space for an expanding mind. A person cannot serve from an empty well. In order to live a life of embodied empathy and compassion, we may have to put a pause on responsibilities so that we may fill our own coffers. This is why coming to the mat in practice feels like coming home: when we tune into the mind-body connection with unfettered attention, we settle into ourselves. We literally come home to the self.

The set of niyamas in Patanjali's *Yoga Sutras* can be seen as an ethical code and prescription for self-care. These guidelines instruct us on how to live from the inside out, how to treat our bodies, how to cultivate room for mental and spiritual growth. It is important that we approach these directives with compassion. Being gentle to ourselves—to forgive ourselves when we do not live up to the standards we've set—is its own form of self-care.

Cancer season is associated with family and memory, and coincides with the summer solstice. The start of summer signifies a homecoming after the frenetic phase of the sun's journey through Gemini. Fiercely protective, Cancerian energy may stimulate a desire to nest. Cancer is symbolized by the Crab—which, of course, carries its home wherever it goes, its hard external shell protecting its soft underbelly. While this nurturing instinct often manifests outwardly as a desire or need to take care of others, it can also be turned inward as a charge to nurture oneself.

PRACTICE

Supine Knee-to-Chest Pose (Apanasana)

Prana is our life force, the energy that moves through us, carried by the breath and nurtured by practice. Apana, conversely, is the release of prana; it is breath moving outward, clearing the body of toxins. Directly translated from Sanskrit as "wind-relieving pose," Knee-to-Chest cleanses the home of our body with vital life force. Begin in Corpse Pose (see page 262) to connect to the ground. Draw one knee to your chest and rock back and forth, and in circular motions around the back of the pelvis, to mitigate tension in your lower back. If there's still residual tightness there, try bending your opposite knee and placing that foot on the ground. The compression of hugging your knee to your chest stimulates the abdominals to improve digestion.

Connection to the earth grounds us into the root (muladhara) chakra, our seat of familial ties and ancestral memory, encouraging a connection to that foundation from which we grow. Our third (solar plexus) chakra is our center of confidence, the power center of self. When we nourish the temple of the body, we create the sense of confidence to go forward into the world.

THIS WEEK: DATE NIGHT FOR ONE

Treat yourself to a date night. Leave your devices at home—a date night with your higher self is not a date night with Instagram!—and take yourself to a restaurant you've been meaning to try, a play you've been wanting to see, or to the park with a small picnic. Make it special: approach this as you would a date night with a loved one. Try not to be distracted or fill the time by reading or listening to music. Instead, listen to the conversations that cycle through your mind. Coming home to yourself is a gift. Self-care is taking the time to be alone and enjoying the comfort of your own company and thoughts in a kind and loving manner.

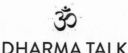

DHARMA TALK

When we return to our roots, to the places
and foundations of family and truth,
we create a home in ourselves;
we nurture courage to grow and to change.
When we tune in and settle
into the home of the heart,
we honor that which feeds the soul
and makes us whole.

RECEPTIVITY

Opening Up to Insight

Each moment presents us with an opportunity to embrace possibility. We get glimpses of these "openings" within a yoga practice: we learn patience as we stumble and fall; we are reminded to honor our limitations. This is how we grow.

Receptivity is the opposite of resistance. Hindu mythology associates receptivity with the feminine and particularly with the goddess Shakti, the divine great mother and archetype for the divine feminine. Her twin flame, Lord Shiva, represents the essence of masculinity. Shakti is the creator and protector, Shiva the destroyer and conqueror. Femininity and masculinity are not intrinsically gendered—we all possess elements of these energies within.

Tantric texts identify the nadis, pathways for energy flowing from root to crown. The ida nadis is our lunar, feminine pathway; pingala is its solar, masculine counterpart. Both are necessary. To teeter too far toward the masculine can cause us to become stuck in detrimental patterns or belief systems. There are indeed times when resistance is necessary, but we must be receptive to those complexities. It is the balance of masculine and feminine, resistance and receptivity, that generates harmony.

Sensory perception is our ability to receive and transmit stimuli through the five senses. We are receptive when we are open and responsive to ideas and suggestions. Perhaps one of the most receptive qualities we have is our ability to listen. When we listen, we inform decisions with what is best for us, our communities, and our planet. But when the ego supersedes, we only listen to what it is we think we want to hear.

Receptivity is dependent upon both our outer and inner impressions. To listen externally is to be attentive and fully present. To listen internally is to convene with the energy of the greater cosmic whole, to lay down our swords and invoke the goddess within.

Receptivity is a trait of Cancer, the zodiac's most feminine sign. Symbolized by the sensitive and compassionate Crab, Cancer is governed by the emotional waters of the tide-pulling moon. When we soften our hard shells and open to what is possible, we receive clarity and insight; we follow the guidance of our intuition. Cancer rules the chest, breast, and abdomen, and, like the Crab, has a delicate underbelly. This invites us to turn inward to hone the loving, nourishing energy that radiates from the heart.

PRACTICE

Reclined Bound Angle Pose
(Supta Baddha Konasana)

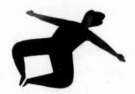

Bound Angle Pose, also known as Cobbler's Pose, was named for the sitting position of cobblers in India. Performed lying down, Reclined Bound Angle Pose facilitates restorative benefits by helping to activate the parasympathetic nervous system, our rest-and-digest response. In yin yoga, this shape, known as Reclined Butterfly, is often supported with props, such as blocks placed beneath the outer knees, for comfort, longevity, and a deeper meditative experience.

Reclined Bound Angle is a hip opener that stretches your groins and inner thighs, and stimulates the abdominal and reproductive organs. This rouses the creative waters of the sacral (svadhisthana) chakra, invoking the fertility of the goddess Shakti to give birth to new ideas. A gentle opening of your chest and heart (anahata) chakra is facilitated by placing the arms wide, grabbing opposite elbows overhead, or drawing your arms into a cactus shape. You may rest your palms on your belly as your internal gaze is directed to the third-eye (ajna) chakra.

THIS WEEK: SURROUND YOURSELF WITH SOUND

In this seated meditation, you will practice receptivity through attentive, effortless listening. Take a comfortable seat that you can sustain for a fifteen-minute duration (optional: set a timer). Notice the myriad layers of sound around you as you hone active listening through effortless awareness. Begin by breathing deeply and noticing the rhythm of your inhales and exhales. Whether you are indoors or outdoors, attune to the sounds around you: the hum of a generator or appliance, the song of birds, or the wind blowing through the trees.

Then allow your attention to drift outward, hearing the frequencies of cars, dogs barking, children laughing, strangers conversing, the reverberation of a neighbor's instrument, and so on—noting, recognizing, and then moving on to the next. Continue quietly observing sound until this action becomes effortless—you're no longer trying, just witnessing and being, noting clarity, wisdom, and insight as it arises.

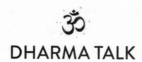

DHARMA TALK

When we listen we convene with the divine
we surrender, we soften, we open, and arrive.
When we are receptive to our innermost silence,
we can hear the hymns of the heart's resonance.

BLOSSOMING

Cultivating Personal Growth

Growth is a negotiation between what you perceive yourself to be and where you see yourself going. Deep spiritual or intellectual work challenges us to look within while remaining anchored through transition. When we connect to our roots, we are able to blossom; like a sprouting seedling, we can only extend upward when we are firmly planted in personal soil. This requires trust and perseverance: we do not always know where we are headed. Sometimes we must traverse through the darkness and discomfort of the vast unknown in order to grow.

In practice, breath is the oxygen; movement the sunshine. Each inhale is an opportunity to create space, each exhale is an opportunity to explore that expansion. The niyama svadhyaya loosely translates as "self-study" and instructs us to find our authentic, whole self by exploring and nurturing our foundations, our beginnings, and our experiences. This may sometimes reveal what we need to let go as much as where we need to focus. A tree sheds its dying leaves to conserve water—consider what may be draining your resources.

Blossoming is a theme that resonates with summer—a time of year when the external world is flush with lush vegetation and blooms.

Much like the insistent seed that bursts forth into a flower, personal growth can only come to fruition through commitment, with sincere introspection and the practice of svadhyaya. A blossoming of the soul gives volume to our capacity.

Blossoming invokes the Cancerian energy that corresponds to our deepest, most sensitive feelings. Watery Cancer is confident that diving into the well of personal and familial truth can yield an emotional and spiritual return on investment. Symbolized by the Crab, Cancer is most at home in itself. Dig deep to find what waters your foundation—but be mindful of Cancerian energy that may cause you to overindulge in nostalgia or blame. What is it that you must weed from your spiritual garden?

PRACTICE

Lotus Pose with Lotus Mudra
(Padmasana)

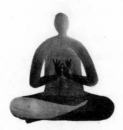

Ancient Buddhist art depicts Lotus Pose as the posture the Buddha, Siddhartha, took while sitting in meditation for seven weeks, which led to his enlightenment under the Bodhi tree. Full Lotus Pose is an advanced seated pose that requires flexibility in the legs and knees, as well as strength in the core. If range of motion is limited in the hips, or the knees are sensitive, try crossing one leg for Half Lotus Pose. If Half Lotus Pose is not accessible, try Easy Seat (Sukhasana; see page 195) as an alternative. Lotus Pose cultivates a strong sense of stability and grounding, allowing you to hold your spine upright. Consistent practice can help to stimulate blood flow in the pelvic region, which may relieve menstrual tension and sciatica pain.

A meditation pose, Lotus engages the root (muladhara) and third-eye (ajna) chakras. The third eye is associated with the moon, the cosmic ruler of Cancer. Drawing your attention to the space between your eyebrows provides a direct lifeline back to your own sense of inner knowing. Lotus Pose is also associated with the opening of the crown (sahasrara) chakra. Symbolized by a thousand-petaled lotus flower, an open and receptive crown chakra is the manifestation of our personal blossoming; of the deep personal work that has allowed us to grow into our fullest potential. Optionally, bring the heels of your palms together, with the thumbs and pinky fingers touching, to form Lotus mudra.

THIS WEEK: NURTURE AFFIRMATIVE BELIEFS

Writing positive affirmations is a useful exercise in honing the qualities and experiences you want to invite in. By turning goals or desires into tangible reminders by writing them out on paper, we welcome them into our reality.

Affirmations can be aspirational (for example, "I've been given the raise I've worked so hard for") or declarative (for example, "I am confident" or "I am beautiful"). It's best to keep affirmations clear, short, and simple—and write them in the present tense as though they've already come true. Place your affirmations in a conspicuous place where you can see them every day, like on the bathroom mirror, as a reminder of what you're nurturing. Affirmations don't only lead to self-development; the power and physical benefit of positive thinking is scientifically proven (John Hopkins Medicine n.d.). Improve your well-being as you blossom.

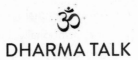

DHARMA TALK

A deep connection to home
gives us the foundation to blossom.
When we look toward the sun
and invite forth the rain,
our souls find nourishment and growth.
Do not be afraid of the mud that
tangles your roots beneath the surface.
Neither forget that even the wettest, darkest night
heralds the promise of warming rays.

PASSION

Stoking the Embers of Your Fire

We are sentient beings propelled by passion. Great wars have been waged, cities have been constructed, and scientific advances have shifted our societal landscape—all in the name of passion, for better or worse. We seek relationships that support our passions as well as like-minded communities that foster a safe space to explore them. When our inner fires are stoked we burn more brightly so that we may radiate that warmth outwardly.

The niyama tapas teaches us to burn away impurities. As the physical world warms up, summer is an opportunity to burn away what we have outgrown; tapas is fire generated by the friction of challenging our routines. By ridding ourselves of excess, we keep ourselves from getting stuck in a rut. When we fail to check in with our actions, we may find ourselves letting life happen to us rather than living intentionally and with integrity.

The practice of sankalpa is the pursuit of a heart-driven resolution that speaks to a specific goal. It is an intention that comes from deep analysis of personal passion, allowing us to pursue that passion without losing control or being overcome by emotion. Just as tapas teaches us to shed, sankalpa helps us to hone actions that align with our integrity. Yoga nidra, or yogic sleep, is a deeply introspective practice for considering sankalpa.

Cancer is the matriarch, the lover and doer of the zodiac. As the first water sign of the zodiac, Cancerian energy is fluid—the stream that starts the flow of creativity. Governed by the moon, Cancerian energy also calls on the center of intuition, our third eye, to channel clear insight around our deepest desires. Ruler of the heart and stomach, Cancer is associated with relationships and the seat of our personal power. Only when that confidence is awakened can we begin to ignite the fires of professional, personal, or creative passion.

PRACTICE

Goddess Pose (Utkata Konasana)

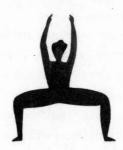

Goddess energy, the creative energy of the universe, is discussed in tantric texts as Shakti energy, the feminine psychospiritual force that balances the masculine Shiva. It can manifest in myriad ways: a call to delve into personal discovery; a call to nurture a deep, honest relationship with the innermost self; a call to live in the pursuit of passion. "Utkata" roughly translates from the Sanskrit as "powerful" or "fierce." Goddess Pose awakens the Shakti energy we all possess.

This empowering pose requires balance and stability, and provides a deep stretch to the inner thighs, hips, and groins. It also engages the core. Heat-building Goddess Pose stimulates and supports good circulation, and it's also a pelvic floor strengthener that may be used in preparation for childbirth.

Goddess Pose stimulates the sacral (svadhisthana) chakra, the center of creativity and sensuality. As the third (manipura) chakra is engaged to support the spinal column, energy can flow more freely. Engagement of this power center bolsters the foundation of our inner reserves as we reconnect to our passions in preparation for the heart-opening cycle of Leo season.

THIS WEEK: SET HEART-CENTERED GOALS

It's easy to get bogged down by daily routine. But when we give ourselves time and space to explore new things to feed our passions, we can explore our ever-evolving sankalpa.

Set aside thirty minutes to an hour and list all the outlandish life goals you remember having as a child. Write them all down—even ones that are completely unrealistic. When your list is finished, consider which still have potential. You may want to alter some. For instance, "Walk on the moon" could become "Experience an antigravity chamber." Or "Be an Oscar-winning actor" could be "Enroll in an acting workshop." Plot each one out on a timeline and choose a few to accomplish. Even if the activity seems like a waste of time, give yourself permission to explore some of the passions that you may have previously written off as foolish.

By navigating discomfort and exploring some of these interests in your adult life, you'll begin to reignite the embers of your inner fire.

DHARMA TALK

There is a fire that does not diminish
despite torrential storms of life.
The lava that bubbles from the core of Earth
is your fiery core too.
It explodes in bits of stardust
we leave in the wake of our truth.
When we have courage to explore what
ignites this fire and makes us whole,
we can share this glow with others.
We become our own guiding light.

VULNERABILITY

The Strength of an Achilles Heel

In a world that has conditioned us to keep our guard up, vulnerability can seem like capitulation. We consider concealing emotion a form of strength, the admittance of shortcomings a weakness. In love, we shield our hearts; at work, we safeguard our ideas. On the mat, we may protect our bodies by avoiding certain postures rather than trying modifications.

To find strength in vulnerability is to understand that even in our most defenseless moments—outside of self-imposed walls—we are not unmoored. We are anchored, supported, and connected to the cosmic whole. The misconception that we are alone and untethered is to be in a state of avidya, which, translated from Sanskrit, means "not knowing," or "the absence of understanding." Vidya, conversely, is understanding that we are tied, inextricably, to the collective unconscious, which gives us deeper, more meaningful purpose.

In practice, we explore vulnerability in physical postures that challenge our bodies by releasing expectations of what those poses "should" look like. When we let go of preconceived notions about perfection, we relearn how to become at ease with where we are. It's not about climbing another rung on the ladder toward advancement. It's about true communion with the self and the interconnected whole. This forces us to recognize unserving patterns—to find comfort within discomfort and bravely navigate the shadowy recesses of the mind. To be vulnerable is to accept our own unique processes.

Vulnerability is a Leo theme, a sign secure in authentic and confident self-expression. Symbolized by the Lion, Leo is a natural-born leader who dares to be vulnerable. Leo energy reminds us that in order to be successful, satisfied, and happy, we cannot hide our truest natures. There is no embarrassment in failure or in the not knowing, only an opportunity to learn and to find connection in vidya. Pitfalls of this sign are often ego related, as Leonine energy compels us to do what we want, when we want—sometimes without consideration of how those actions may affect others.

PRACTICE

Crescent Lunge (Anjaneyasana)

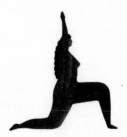

Anjaneyasana is named for the mother of the Monkey God Lord Hanuman, Anjani, and the shape of a young child reaching in devotion toward the sun.

Stabilizing the pelvis and targeting the deep core muscles engages the transverse abdominis to facilitate a slight backbend. This helps stimulate the flow of prana in an upward motion along the spinal cord. Crescent Lunge, also called Low Lunge, stretches the hip flexors while engaging the quadriceps and glutes. To avoid overstretching the psoas and "dumping" into the shape, emphasize the rootedness of this posture from the waist down, lifting up and out of the lumbar. Lengthen both sides of your body and create more spaciousness in between the ribs. Pressing your front foot into the earth helps to stabilize the hips.

Leo is ruled by the sun and corresponds to the heart, chest, thoracic spine, and upper back. By strengthening the core and hips, this pose taps into the third (manipura) chakra, our energetic power center, building confidence. The natural backbend encourages the opening of the heart (anahata) chakra to embrace vulnerability from a place of compassion.

THIS WEEK: WRITE AN OLD-FASHIONED LETTER

Dare to express how you truly feel to someone in your life by way of a written letter. Choose to write to someone with whom you have not spoken recently. It doesn't have to be long; simply telling someone you love or forgive them is one of the most vulnerable things you can do. The act of writing—of using pen and paper to relay your thoughts rather than by digital proxy—evokes vulnerability because it requires the transmission of one's emotional energy into physical space, untainted by electronic 1s and 0s.

This practice helps to cultivate more gratitude in your relationships and allows you to release unhealthy emotions. Being vulnerable through the ways we communicate creates space for new relationships and experiences.

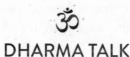

DHARMA TALK

We are not floating blindly, untethered.
We are as interconnected as the roots to leaves,
as the cycles of the moon pulling on sea.
Grounded as we are to
blood, breath,
love, memory—
how can we ever be lost?
The fear we release
and the peace that we chase—
it has been within us all along.

HUMILITY

Who We Are Underneath It All

Healthy competition drives innovation and advancement. Unhealthy competition is evidenced by a constant need to push and prove our value and worthiness—even on the mat. In all things, but particularly when it comes to mindfulness practices, humility paves the way to advancement and achievement.

Humans are socialized to take seriously the pursuit of our ambitions. We value that which may determine or validate our identities; our appearances establish self-importance. The sutras describe the koshas as energetic facades or sheaths behind which we conceal our true selves. These layers represent both self-perception and how we wish to be perceived. To recognize that self-importance is a false longing of the ego is to peel back those sheaths, remove the masks, and dissolve the facades.

When we embrace humility through this uneasy process of unspooling, we channel our innate genuineness. We amplify who it is we truly are through the raw and tender honesty that emanates from the heart. As narcissism fades into a dark, spiraling pool of unshackled vanity and self-righteousness, we are liberated from the limiting beliefs of the stories we carry—and with it the heavy burdens that place the weight of the world on our shoulders.

The lightheartedness of summertime invites us to swap serious-
ness with pleasure. When self-consciousness looms over self-confidence, we are incapable of experiencing this joy. Laughing at our
limitations reminds us of what it means to be human.

We can practice humility during Leo season, an expressive, heartfelt
cycle famous for its Lion's pride. Leo is a fire sign ruled by the sun,
the largest star in our solar system that gives us life, the light from
which naturally boosts confidence and esteem. When the illusion of
pride shrouds us from the truth, this veil acts like a sheath of armor
to protect our vulnerable hearts. Associated with the chest, spine, and
upper back, Leo empowers us to lead from the heart. By operating
from the heart-brain—our cardiac nervous system of neurotransmitters—we can send the heart's messages to the brain in pursuit of our
passions.

PRACTICE

Humble Warrior (Baddha Virabhadrasana)

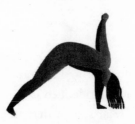

Humble Warrior, also called Devotional Warrior, stretches the shoulders, strengthens the back muscles, mobilizes the thoracic spine, and opens the chest and heart (anahata) chakra. To avoid straining your knees, take a shorter and wider stance to hone the strength of your legs. Maintain optimal range of motion in the shoulder extensors (latissimus dorsi, a.k.a. lats) by bending at your elbows to stabilize the triceps.

This shape tones the abdominal muscles and activates the solar plexus (manipura) chakra to sustain your purpose, humor, and wit, as the ego is said to be forged within these proverbial fires. Humble Warrior is a bowing to the divine. Any yoga posture that puts the head below the heart can help to fire the heart-brain neurotransmitters. This regulates function of the pineal gland, the small endocrine gland that balances hormones and produces melatonin to manage circadian rhythms, located between the two cerebral hemispheres in the brain. In doing so, the third-eye (ajna) chakra is opened.

THIS WEEK: TRY LAUGHTER AS MEDICINE

Laughter is the first step toward making the spiritual shift toward humility—especially when the ego defines something as stupid, embarrassing, or shameful. Not everyone has the ability to laugh at their shortcomings, but a study found that those who were able to laugh at themselves had a more jovial personality—revealing a link between hilarity and humility (Beermann and Ruch 2011).

Turn back the clock to one of the most embarrassing moments of your life. Are you still cringing in humiliation or pretending like it never happened? Let the moment come to mind and grant yourself permission to relive it. This time, give yourself the gift of a big, hearty Buddha-belly laugh. To laugh at our limitations is to practice radical self-love in its purest, most primal form. With enough practice, it becomes possible to laugh at ourselves even when we make the most cringe-worthy of mistakes. This is a means of taking back our power from any perceived judgment and ridicule from others, and especially any judgment or ridicule that stems directly from ourselves. It is the backbone of a humble, embodied self.

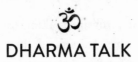

DHARMA TALK

What lies beneath
the masks and the sheaths?
What is hidden by the
identities we cling to?
Nothing is below you
just as nothing is above.
Never mind your ego,
just do the work.
When the heart and mind are full,
you have all that you need.

EXPRESSION

Speaking Your Truth

To embark on a spiritual journey to realize your fullest expression is to explore jñānamarga, the path of classical yoga that emphasizes knowledge and discovery. We all have a unique purpose to serve in this life. Yet truth—and the expression of it—is not solely an internal task. When we begin to understand who we are, we can come to fully appreciate our unique gifts and share them outwardly. Satya is the yama that asks us to examine the way we speak, to consider whether our actions, words, and deeds are within our individual integrity. Satya asks us to reconcile our internal personal truth with the way we express ourselves externally.

Embodying satya on the mat is to allow practice to be exactly what it is in the moment—to surrender, gracefully, to the here and now. How does the pose feel? What are you experiencing? Your satya in your practice is to not push past your edge but to honor your process. What are your personal boundaries? How do you show up for your body and yourself in an effort to explore them?

A fixed fire sign, Leo is one of the most expressive archetypes of the zodiac. Leo is associated with strong leadership and pride (sometimes to the point of fault), but Leonine energy also teaches us how to embody personal power through honorable, noble expression. During Leo season, we can channel the steadfast Lion to turn impossible dreams into tangible reality. Finding our own truth—whether through self-discovery in the jñāna tradition or by examining how we externally engage—is what provides a sense of immutability in a constantly changing world.

PRACTICE

Upward-Facing Dog
(Urdhva Mukha Svanasana)

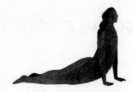

The name for this posture is derived from the Sanskrit words "urdhva," which translates to "up," and "mukha," meaning "face." In the Mahabharata, there is a story of the Pandava brothers. Upon arrival in heaven, Indra told Yudhisthira that his dog could not accompany him. Citing the dog's loyalty, Yudhisthira refused to abandon him; the dog was revealed to be Yudhisthira's godfather, and Yudhisthira was rewarded. Upward-Facing Dog is a reminder of devotion to the expression of personal truth.

Leo governs the heart, spine, and upper back. Upward Dog stretches the trapezius muscles, responsible for movement and stabilization of the shoulder blades. In this backbend, the back of your neck (the cervical spine) extends to help open your throat and chest. Maintain space between your ears and shoulders by keeping a slight bend in the elbows. Be wary of collapsing into your lower back, overarching your neck, or dropping your head back, which compresses the cervical spine.

Upward Dog opens the heart (anahata) chakra as the chest broadens. As the throat (vishuddha) chakra is stimulated, we can speak our truths with more confidence. By drawing focus toward the third-eye (ajna) chakra—associated with the sun, the ruling planet of Leo—we learn to draw from quiet intuition and wisdom. That is the seat and the expression of satya.

THIS WEEK: DISCOVER YOUR PERSONAL TRUTHS

We are multifaceted creatures with seemingly disparate goals and paths. How do we discover our personal truths and then live in the integrity of them? The first step is to reflect on the beliefs that make you who you are.

Fill in the blanks for the following sentences:

I believe in _____.

I am worthy of _____.

I love to _____.

I enjoy _____.

I dislike doing _____.

My favorite memory last year was _____.

Then, for one week, keep a log of your activities and include notes about any significant happenings. At the end of the week, analyze which activities—or feelings about them—were in accordance with the above sentences. How are you expressing your innermost truths? What could shift so that your routines stay aligned with your truths? Express your satya loud and proud, much like the noble Lion.

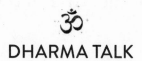

DHARMA TALK

Your innate truth
binds you to the greater world,
propels you toward your fullest potential.
This expression binds you to the planet
no different than secrets on the wind,
than energy lapped by frothing waves,
than the fragrant musk of crawling soil.
Your truth is as integral as moondust.
You have a right to be here.

LOVE

Embracing All That You Are

Epigenetics, the study of genetic memory, examines how memories from previous generations are passed on through shared DNA structures. These cellular impressions manifest as prodigious, unexplained talents, but they also appear as trauma, fear, or anxiety. What if some of these cellular inheritances were responsible for the common inability to love ourselves? Not only is our inner critic an unreliable narrator, it's also a byproduct of a lineage of negative thinking from our predecessors. Perhaps we inherit our karma after all.

The path toward self-love is one of devotion, or bhakti, of fondness and faith. In Hinduism, the practice of bhakti is based on the worship of a god or deity. The teachings of bhakti, however, can be incorporated into modern life without doctrine or dogma, just as the Buddhist principle of contentment can be applied to contemporary thinking without adhering to ideology.

The Buddha described love as total spiritual liberation; it is universal love that completes us—not another person. Divine love is infinite, beyond the limitations of social complexities. When we practice this form of love, the hardened heart begins to soften as impurities of the mind melt away. The neural pathways of gestational memories that germinated into consciousness are slowly rewired after lifetimes on the fritz. By rewriting these conditionings, we experience greater empathy and compassion toward ourselves and one another.

But love does not always come easy. Whether inherited or habituated, we may spend a lifetime unlearning the patterns that prevented us from truly loving ourselves as we are; from realizing that real love is always available to us. At our innermost source, we are, after all, only love. Perfectly imperfect, raw, messy, devotional love.

Love falls in the domain of Leo's noble Lion, the zodiac's proud and passionate sign. Leo is governed by the sun, which fuels our purpose and ego. If we operate too much from this proverbial power center, however, we subconsciously mute the heart's messages. To heal our psyche, we must learn how to listen, rekindle our passions and desires, and heed our heart's highest calling. Ruler of the chest, spine, and upper back, the fierce Leonine archetype can be called on to target the heart as we practice the art of loving ourselves.

PRACTICE

Reverse Warrior
(Viparita Virabhadrasana)

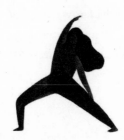

Reverse Warrior, also called Exalted Warrior or Peaceful Warrior, is a gesture of opening to all that is coming—an offering of the heart as love is radiated inwardly and outwardly. This posture stretches the chest, shoulders, and upper arms; mobilizes the thoracic spine; lengthens the torso; and strengthens the abdominal wall. The ankles, quadriceps, and glutes engage to stabilize the hips. By bringing a microbend to your back knee, weight can be distributed between your front and back legs more evenly.

The gaze, or drishti, is focused toward the fingertips reaching overhead, awakening the third-eye (ajna) chakra. The heart (anahata) chakra is opened to allow messages to flow from the heart to the pineal gland. The solar plexus (manipura) chakra is also activated, empowering you to utilize your innate gifts in conjunction with the desires of the heart.

THIS WEEK: A LETTER FROM THE WOUNDED HEALER

Spend some time in quiet, contemplative inquiry with a rose quartz crystal. Consider the possibility that any lack of self-love or self-worth you might possess could stem from your ancestral heritage, your past, or a core childhood wound. If a specific memory comes to mind, painful as it may be, allow whatever feelings, sensations, or thoughts that percolate to come to the surface—tempting as it may be to resist and stuff them back down. Breathe deeply, reciting the mantra "Aham prema" ("I am divine love") and cultivating compassion toward yourself as you reflect.

Next, write a letter to your younger self. What would you want this younger version of you to know? This process, though difficult, is cathartic, healing, and deeply moving. Write from the perspective of the wounded healer. Consider that maybe you, your parents, their parents, their grandparents, and so on, have been sharing genetic memory or unhealed karmic lessons. Utilize the teachings of your past trauma(s) to begin, or continue, the process of healing your heart. Loving yourself despite your flaws, and forgiving those who have hurt you (despite theirs), is the gateway toward healing your subconscious by way of your heart and attaining emotional independence.

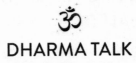

DHARMA TALK

Love is a kaleidoscopic spectrum
radiating prismatic layers
and emitting frequencies from the heart.
Love begins with acceptance
and culminates with compassion.
When we love ourselves
and are kind to ourselves,
we learn to love and be kind to one another.
Only love is infinite; only love is real.

JOY

Celebrating Life

We tend to wait for special occasions to give ourselves permission to celebrate. Yet every moment is an opportunity to celebrate life. Even the simplest, most automatic of body functions, like breathing, is a tiny miracle happening in and around us each day.

Joy often manifests as happiness, but happiness is fleeting. Joy is a state of being that comes from within. In the Bhagavad Gita, the highest of the three gunas (threads of existence), sattva, is defined as harmony, joy, and intelligence (Easwaran 2007). We experience sattva when we release expectations of finding it externally. We all possess the potential for joy within.

Life is full of trying or tragic moments during which finding joy may seem impossible. We can choose not to let ourselves become ensnared by mundane struggles or stressors. No emotion—regardless how high or low, or light or dark, it may be—is invalid, but problems arise when we focus on the negative. Brilliant as the mind may be, it is its nature to fixate on problems. The nature of the soul is to counteract those negative tendencies: to spark joy, create, regenerate, and seek out the good in everything and everyone.

When we forget how to enjoy ourselves and those around us, we operate on a lower energetic frequency. By attuning to the higher frequency of love, we are reminded that life is too short to *not* be enjoyed. Even the smallest shift in a mindset can make any moment more tolerable—and maybe even a little magical. Joy is always available to us, bubbling just below the surface, boundless and infinite.

Ruled by the sun, Leo is bold and passionate, and though the energy of this fire sign can be egomaniacal, it encourages fearless pursuit of dreams. Leo is associated with the chest and spine, and, much like the courageous Lion, proudly wears its heart on a sleeve. The zodiac's eternal child, Leo is filled with wonder, reminding us of our innate playful natures that we leave behind as we transition to adulthood. Inviting our inner child out to play is the rediscovery of joy and pleasure, and our existence becomes a celebration of a life well lived.

PRACTICE

Wild Thing
(Camatkarasana)

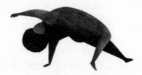

Wild Thing, also called Rock Star Pose, has been described as "the ecstatic unfolding of the enraptured heart." It's an invigorating, enlivening posture that opens our hearts to unfettered joy. It is rare to see a frown or furrowed brow on a yogi actively exploring this pose; even the name, Wild Thing, begets a smile.

This shape mobilizes the thoracic spine by opening the chest and upper back, and it stretches the shoulder girdle. Hip flexors lengthen while the quadriceps strengthen, and there is a sense of playfulness as the whole world is turned upside down. Entering the shape from in between Downward-Facing Dog (see page 214) and Plank Pose (see page 210) helps you flip yourself over with more safety, stability, and ease. By extending through the crown of your head, your gaze will naturally follow your palm as it reaches overhead.

Wild Thing helps facilitate the heart-to-head transmission of information, activating the pineal gland to rouse the third-eye (ajna) chakra. The pose helps unblock the throat (vishuddha) chakra, encouraging unabashed self-expression from a place of truth. A tremendous heart-opener, Wild Thing creates spaciousness to make room for joy.

THIS WEEK: IMPROMPTU DANCE PARTY

If yoga is a dance of the soul, dancing is the self illuminated. Studies have shown that dancing can reduce stress and help alleviate depression and anxiety (Akandere and Demir 2011; Lesté and Rust 1984); the act of shaking the body releases endorphins that melt away tension and promote relaxation. Dance makes us more resilient, helping us live longer and with more vitality. Dancing is cathartic, creative, and healing.

Treat yourself to a private dance party for one. Put on your favorite song and shake off what no longer serves you. Much like your yoga practice, don't worry about how it looks; focus instead on how it *feels*. Let your movement flow naturally, organically, rhythmically, and intuitively. Dance like you were born to, and dance like there's no tomorrow—because all we really have anyway is right now. And right now is indeed something to celebrate.

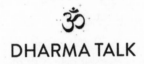

DHARMA TALK

Life is a celebration
to enjoy, and be joyous
here and now.
A life well lived is to remember
that every breath we take,
that every morning we wake,
we have been given an incredible gift—
one to celebrate, to honor, to enjoy.

23

PURIFICATION

The Discipline of Refinement

Purity is associated with austerity, a renunciation of worldly pleasures. In the Judeo-Christian context, purity connotes celibacy or denial of hedonism—choices that some may find unrealistic. On the opposite end of extremes is a reckless blind hunger to indulge in libertine pursuits. As with all things, purity is about balance and moderation.

Saucha is the first principle of self-discipline in the five niyamas, translated as "purification" or "cleanliness." The sutras teach that by keeping the body clean, our emotions mirror a clearer inner self. The practice of saucha illuminates our truest, most joyful natures.

We experience saucha through asana (cultivating a healthy physical body), pranayama (purification of the energetic body), and tapas. Tapas is the self-discipline of burning away the patterns that no longer serve us. The *Hatha Yoga Pradipika* (Mohan 2017), a fifteenth-century text that elucidates the science of hatha yoga, outlines the practice of saucha through six cleansing techniques known as shatkarma.

Traditional shatkarma may not seem entirely practical, though we can still understand the directive in modern application. The choices we make around diet, mind-altering substances, and the products we use are all pragmatic functions of saucha. While there is much debate in the yoga world regarding whether to eat meat or drink alcohol, on the flipside, too much deprivation can lead to orthorexia, a condition that centers around obsessive healthy eating. When part of a balanced system, saucha is to fine-tune or polish the soul.

When we have burned away what is unnecessary, we realize enjoyment and pleasure free of distraction. Saucha is to live purely and to discover fulfillment within the choices we make.

Symbolized by the Virgin, a maiden carrying a shaft of wheat, earth-sign Virgo shifts our attention to cleaner living and prioritizing well-being. Ruled by Mercury, planet of communication, Virgo energy is environmentally conscious and feminine, encouraging grace and refinement. It is associated with the digestive system and intestinal tract, gallbladder, spleen, pancreas, and the nervous system. Virgo's glyph is an M, meant to represent the intestines or virginity.

PRACTICE

Crescent Lunge with a Twist
(Anjaneyasana Variation)

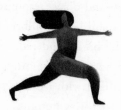

Anjaneyasana is named for Hanuman's mother, Anjani. It is considered a devotional pose, symbolic of a person reaching toward the heavens.

This standing twist is a functional take on a Revolved Crescent Lunge (Parivrtta Anjaneyasana), in which hands are brought together in front of the heart and spine is torqued to draw elbow to opposite knee. Bring ease to this modification by remaining upright and extending your arms out wide. By finding rotation from the rib cage, Crescent Lunge with a Twist widens the wingspan to open the chest and shoulders. It is often speculated that twisting postures help stimulate digestion and wring out impurities as blood flow circulates to the internal organs and kidneys, though there's not really any hard science to back up those claims.

Turning the chin slightly opens the throat (vishuddha) chakra, so long as you avoid over-rotation in your neck (cervical spine). As the internal organs are stimulated, the solar plexus (manipura) chakra becomes activated. Spaciousness cultivated in the back body between the shoulder blades as well as in the chest facilitates an opening of the heart (anahata) chakra.

Cancer Leo Virgo

THIS WEEK: SEATED MEDITATION WITH ALTERNATE SIDE NOSTRIL BREATHING (NADI SHODHANA)

Nadi shodhana pranayama ("subtle energy-clearing breathing technique") activates the rest-and-digest response of the parasympathetic nervous system. It reestablishes equilibrium between the left and right hemispheres of the brain, and reduces stress and anxiety. As toxins are released and hormones are brought into balance, respiratory channels are revitalized with fresh oxygen, which can improve breathing and alleviate allergy symptoms.

This technique is practiced by alternating between plugging the right nostril (surya nadi) and the left nostril (chandra nadi)—or, in other words, the sun and the moon. Take a comfortable, cross-legged Easy Seat (Sukhasana; see page 195). Rest your left hand in your lap as you sit upright. Place your right index and middle fingers at the third eye, and plug the left nostril with your ring finger as you breathe in through the right nostril. Pause, then plug the right nostril with your thumb and release the right ring finger, exhaling with a cleansing breath out the left nostril. Plug the left nostril again as you breathe in through the right; plug the left nostril again as you exhale through the left. Continue breathing rhythmically for one to five minutes, depending on your level of experience.

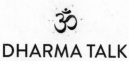

DHARMA TALK

Our bodies are home to a soul,
to divine bits of stardust
gleaming through word and deed.
When this vessel is clean,
our intentions are connected
and our minds are protected.
Clarity within mirrors clarity without.

24

SIMPLIFICATION

When Order Is in Order

It's easy to overcomplicate life. But when the every day starts to feel like it's become crazy busy, it's as much a reflection of the outer landscape as the inner. Simplifying requires us to pare down overscheduled calendars, make time for self-care, and carve out space to breathe and just be. This may mean saying no when we might usually say yes, or decluttering and reorganizing our homes or offices. In so doing, we develop more manageable routines and create healthier habits, and may even learn how to ask for support.

Sometimes to simplify we need to go back to the basics: sit in quiet, contemplative inquiry and observe sensation as it arises. In practice, this could mean placing less emphasis on complicated sequencing, fancy postures, or the "fullest expression of a pose." We practice yoga asana for the sake of practice alone, without ego-driven goals of advancement. Yoga may be ancient, but the poses themselves are not. The word "asana," which literally translates to "a seat," was once the only posture ever practiced for those who sought inner peace.

Virgo season is a time for boosting efficiency, for stripping away excess and prioritizing self-improvement. As the sign of the Virgin ruled by Mercury, the meticulous planet of communication, Virgo is a perfectionist. This methodical energy helps us invite in order and simplicity to the messy and chaotic corners of our lives. Virgo is also known for being a people pleaser and tends to serve everyone but themselves. Be wary of the resentment this may cause.

PRACTICE

Legs Up the Wall
(Viparita Karani)

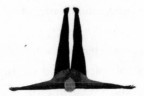

Legs Up the Wall is a restorative posture that is an ideal substitute for Shoulder Stand (Salamba Sarvangasana; see page 52), since it does not place weight on the neck. Classical Hindu yoga texts describe the upward-moving energy, or kundalini, through the spinal cord that an inversion such as this can facilitate.

As one of the most effective postures to ease discomfort in the lower back, Legs Up the Wall stimulates the rest-and-digest state of the parasympathetic nervous system. It's a gentle stretch to relieve foot, leg, or menstrual cramps. It also helps to regulate blood pressure, reduce anxiety, alleviate headaches, and even mitigate symptoms of mild depression (Lee 2010; Zickl 2017; *Gaia* staff n.d.). If tension arises in the lifted legs, bring your feet together and let your knees fall out wide, or let your legs release into a straddle against the wall.

Legs Up the Wall retains the natural curvature in the cervical spine, which helps to open the throat (vishuddha) chakra. The spine rests in neutral to stimulate the root (muladhara) chakra, at the base of the tailbone, up to the crown (sahasrara) chakra. When the arms are held wide or in a cactus shape, the front of the body broadens to open the heart (anahata) chakra. The internal gaze can focus on the space between the brows, the third-eye (ajna) chakra, in self-inquiry and reflection.

THIS WEEK: DECLUTTER YOUR CLOSET

Choice adds value to our lives—but the burden of having an abundance of choices can actually lead to a sense of emptiness. Having too much clutter in our lives feels heavy and distracting, and even disrupts the flow of creativity. Marie Kondo's widely popular book, *The Life-Changing Magic of Tidying Up,* describes the Japanese art of feng shui as a way to improve energy flow within the home. If our outer world is a reflection of our inner, then a cluttered home mirrors a cluttered mind. Think of how much lighter you've felt any time you've done a good cleanout and set aside things to donate, sell, or recycle. In a consumerist culture that values material possessions, it is easy to forget that experiences are far more rewarding.

Go through your closet and pull out anything you have not worn in the last two years (if not less). Unless these items are prized family heirlooms or formal attire you might wear again, dispose of them mindfully. Notice what comes up during this process. Observe when you try to talk yourself out of letting go of something. Note any tension that arises. Once you've finished, notice whether you feel energetically lighter.

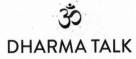

DHARMA TALK

How easy it is
to get caught up in doing and to forget about being,
to take the beauty of the ordinary for granted.
When we realize the serenity of simplicity,
the most mundane tasks become sacred.
Fulfillment lies in the simple—
untangled from webs of complexity.
When we uncomplicate
we create more space
to breathe.

RESPONSIBILITY

To Be in the Service of Others

Responsibility can feel like a burden, dictating how our time and energy is spent. Worse, it becomes conflated with fear of criticism or culpability. With great responsibility, however, comes great joy. To hold oneself accountable is an admittance of self-competence, nourishing a strong sense of self. When we live a life in service, we take pleasure in sharing our unique gifts and foster feelings of contentment.

Karma yoga, one of the four yogic paths, is the path of selfless service, of seva. It dictates that there is no reward, no quid pro quo, no expectation of recognition. In ancient India, the act of seva was considered a step toward spiritual enlightenment. Enlightenment, however, isn't the "goal," just as spiritual fulfillment in practice doesn't come from getting "better" at yoga.

When it comes to service, it is our responsibility to remain authentic and avoid the slippery slope of a savior complex. Selfless service is rooted in a genuine desire to help others without ego. It is not colonial volunteerism. Is that where the work is truly needed—or are you projecting solutions without taking the time to fully understand that need? Beginning a seva practice is an exercise in remaining humble—and then finding joy within that humility.

Responsibility and duty are associated with the energy of Virgo. Ruled by Mercury, the planet of communication, Virgo reminds us that active listening is a requirement for service. Ancient cultures linked the constellation of Virgo—a sign symbolized by the Maiden, carrying a shaft of wheat—to agriculture, associating late summer with preparations for harvest. A sense of responsibility during this cycle is rooted deep within the fertile soil of our collective past.

The Yoga Almanac

PRACTICE

Seated Forward Fold
(Paschimottanasana)

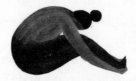

Seated Forward Fold increases circulation to the liver and kidneys, as well as to the uterus, making it a potential relief for menstrual discomfort. As the base of the seat is anchored, the knees can bend slightly to facilitate a hinging at the hips. Consider placing a rolled-up blanket beneath your knees.

To fold into yourself is humbling. When you come into a Seated Forward Fold, you are bowing not only to yourself but honoring your small yet significant place in this world—a crucial sentiment in seva. This pose activates the root (muladhara) chakra by releasing into gravity. As the neck releases, the throat (vishuddha) chakra may open gently. The posture also stimulates the solar plexus (manipura) chakra, our center of outward action and empowerment.

THIS WEEK: GIVE BACK

While donating money to a nonprofit is one form of charitable responsibility, the challenge here is to selflessly donate *yourself* and your time. Seva does not happen at arm's length, regardless of intention. Again, it's about the release of the ego, which, in this sense, manifests as a willingness to place the needs of others above personal schedules or availability constraints.

Stock shelves in a soup kitchen, weed a community garden, organize a volunteer day with your employer, or offer your talents to a local nonprofit. Because Virgo is ruled by Mercury, the planet of communication, flex your interpersonal muscles: ask a charity what it needs the most help with.

But of course, life is busy. There are other ways to ritualistically make seva a part of your life, even if you do not have extra hours in the week to volunteer. You can anonymously pick up the grocery bill or coffee tab for the person in line behind you. Random acts of kindness are seva in action when they're given intentionally and not performatively.

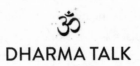

DHARMA TALK

Service need not be a burden.
Responsibility is the thread that binds us
in the great skein of humanity.
To listen, to hear, and to act
toward the freedom of another
is to manifest an egoless existence.
It is to find one's own happiness
in the happiness of others
to recognize our cosmic connection.

26

CONTENTMENT

Becoming at Ease with What Is

To be at peace does not necessitate the absence of chaos, confusion, or stress. It necessitates a sense of calm in the storm. Yoga is not just a respite from the demands of day-to-day life. Practice is a tool to navigate life's challenges from a place of stability, a foundation for living from the heart with ease.

Santosha is the niyama that, more than a directive to "be happy," teaches the practice of contentment. It asks us to do our best with whatever the task may be and to be okay with the outcome—even when that result is unintended or unexpected. Practice helps liberate the mind from reactionary thinking.

We may desire a yoga practice to increase strength and flexibility, or have the expectation of mastering inversions and arm balances. In a social-media-driven world where contortionism is rewarded with attention, hypermobility is conflated with flexibility, which can lead to injury. This isn't yoga. A yogi acknowledges individual progress, knowing when to slow down and back off, and when it's safe to explore. This is described in a yoga practice as the difference between observable sensation and pain. Through the language of movement, we identify where our boundaries lie by honoring both our abilities and limitations. To practice santosha on the mat is to resist muddying the discipline of practice with the expectation of progress.

The idea of being content with our circumstances can feel foreign in a world driven by measurable achievement—but contentment is not complacency. By releasing ourselves from expectations surrounding outcome, we more readily accept where we're at on the journey.

Virgo season is an apt time to discuss contentment, as Virgo energy is analytical and meticulous, known for being obsessive. This season may be an overly critical time, be it of ourselves or others. As a grounded earth sign, however, the meticulousness of Virgo shifts our attention toward clean living and well-being. By practicing contentment during a cycle when we are being hard on ourselves and each other, we are reminded that there is more to life than perfection.

PRACTICE

Seated Spinal Twist
(Marichyasana III)

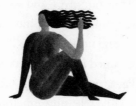

"Marichi" is loosely translated as "sage" or "a ray of light from the sun or moon." Marichi is the son of Brahma and one of seven seers (rishis), or lords of creation (prajapatis). Marichi is also the great-grandfather of Manu, who, in Vedic tradition, is considered the father of the human race.

Seated Spinal Twist, also known as Sage's Pose or Marichi's Pose, stimulates the abdominal organs. When we tend to this "second brain," we create clarity and alleviate nervousness, aiding the body's natural detoxification process. The posture benefits a healthy spine when rotation is natural and not forced.

Seated Spinal Twist rouses the root (muladhara) chakra and taps into our place of personal peace. Tuning into our sacral (svadhisthana) chakra—the center of our creativity—allows us to hone what makes us tick, what helps us feel centered and whole. A slight turn of the chin will open the throat (vishuddha) chakra to increase our ability to communicate from a place of serenity and calm.

THIS WEEK: GROUND THYSELF

Spending time in nature boosts our immune system, improves mood, accelerates recovery from injury or illness, increases energy levels, and, of course, improves sleep (Williams 2017). Mindfulness meditation asks that we observe ourselves and our surroundings in the present moment so that we may become more at ease with what is.

Go for a nature walk and notice the small things we so easily take for granted. Be it the untamed forest or a city park, observe the environment around you. Pay attention to your breath and feel sensation arise within your body, while releasing attachment from the outcome of your stroll. Even the most basic activity, such as an afternoon walk, can become sacred when it is infused with palpable presence and attention. We become more at ease and more capable of accepting ourselves in the moment. This is the practice of contentment.

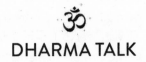

DHARMA TALK

We do not strive for contentment
but create space for it to enter.
Contentment is not complacency
but finding strength in simplicity
and power in the peaceful.
By softening, accepting,
and releasing what is not,
we establish inner peace
and find ease with what is.

AUTUMN

Embracing Transition and Finding Equilibrium

Libra ● Scorpio ● Sagittarius

All this is full. All that is full.

From fullness, fullness comes.

When fullness is taken from fullness,

Fullness still remains.

—The Upanishads

Autumn is a transitional season, straddling the ripeness of summer and the scarcity of winter. It's a time to slow down and regain equilibrium in a rushed world. Here, we may contemplate our needs in relation to others and create routines that encourage a sense of fullness.

As the leaves change and the globe begins to tilt on its axis away from the warmth of the sun, we too take stock of where we are and where we're going. The levity of summer fades into busy, hectic routines—school starts again and we usher in the holiday season—making autumn a time for grounding into practices and habits that generate a sense of balance and harmony. Even as we celebrate the fruition of summer's harvest in the early days of autumn, as days become shorter and colder we may find ourselves experiencing a sense of loss as we navigate this transitory phase. Exploring themes of duality, of light and dark, reminds us how to find stability even as the world keeps turning.

The autumnal equinox marks the first day of Libra season, occurring around September 22 or 23 each year. Libra is the seventh sign of the zodiac wheel and is associated with relationships and peace-keeping. It's ruled by the love planet Venus, which is associated with the heart (anahata) chakra. In order to effectively embrace transition, we must operate from a place of true loving-kindness toward ourselves and others.

Then comes Scorpio season, beginning around October 23, which is ruled by Pluto, the planet of power and transformation. The intensity of Scorpio urges us to navigate our shadow sides and traverse the darker aspects of the self in order to reemerge from the flames. Scorpio is associated with the solar plexus (manipura) chakra, the seat of our personal power.

Sagittarius season commences November 21 or 22 and winds down the last four weeks of the autumnal cycle before winter begins. Ruled by Jupiter, the planet of luck and good fortune, Sagittarius energy invites us to move forward into the rawness of winter from a place of faith and optimism. Sagittarius is associated with the pleasure-seeking sacral (svadhisthana) chakra, the font of creativity and passion.

Autumn is both pitta and vata season in Ayurveda. The early days of autumn, around harvest, are still characterized by the heat of pitta—which, in the Northern Hemisphere, we identify as "Indian summer." Around the autumnal equinox, we may still feel pulled toward the cooling practices we began during summer. By midautumn, as the weather begins to shift, we transition to vata season. Vata energy, characterized by the air element, has qualities of change and movement, and can spur a restlessness of spirit in transition.

In Native American medicine wheel traditions, autumn is associated with the West. It is a time for the death (or hibernation) of vegetation, encouraging deep introspection inside the metaphorical dark cave of the mind. The totem animal of the West is a bear—a powerful, fierce archetype that teaches us to stand strong in the face of loss or evolution. Autumn requires us to find our footing and bravely dive inward, as we let old parts of ourselves fall away in preparation for the introspective season of winter to come.

27

BALANCE

The Dualistic Nature of Reality

Each year at the autumnal equinox, we recognize the symmetry between light and dark, as Mother Nature establishes equilibrium between day and night. As Earth's Northern Hemisphere tilts away from the warmth of the sun, we turn our attention inward for the slower, darker, and colder months to come. What was once flourishing and alive begins its annual process of release and renewal. Much like the inherent duality of all things, we may find ourselves yearning for inner and outer balance this season.

We seek balance in our personal and professional relationships, in our career and home life, and in our minds and bodies. As fall can be a frenetic time of year, there is a need for grounding, a moment for stabilization amid the frenzy. This sense of evenness is described in Sanskrit as samatva or samata: a state of inner peace, harmony, and balance.

We move and rest, work and play, succeed and fail, celebrate and grieve, create and destroy. It is within this yoking that we develop an understanding that the dark and light, the difficult and easy, must coexist together. As we rise above to non-duality, we awaken to greater insight and clarity—despite the chaos and commotion that swirls below.

The first day of fall—the autumnal equinox—coincides with the start of Libra season. As the seventh sign of the zodiac, Libra is associated with committed partnerships and marks a time for inviting balance back to body and mind after the whirlwind of summer. Symbolized by the Scales of Justice, always weighing the good and bad, Libra season is when we hone the harmonious qualities of this air sign and invite more peace into our lives. With Venus, the planet of beauty and equity, as Libra's cosmic ruler, we are also reminded to strive for healthy emotional independence within our relationships.

PRACTICE

Half Moon Pose
(Ardha Chandrasana)

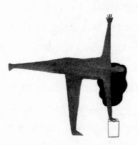

Balancing postures serve as a bridge between earth and air to reestablish inner and outer equilibrium. Balancing strengthens muscles and ligaments to prevent injury as well as sharpens our reflexes. Half Moon Pose balances two opposing forces by channeling the energies of lunar calm and solar fire. By grounding into your center of serenity and extending outwardly, you become more relaxed and at ease—despite the physical challenges of the shape. By yoking moon and sun, you essentially transcend from that dyad and get a glimpse at non-duality.

Half Moon strengthens and tones the glutes, legs, and ankles, as well as opens the hips and groins. Libra rules the lumbar region, and this pose can ask for a lot of effort from the lower back. To strengthen the lower back muscles, Half Moon can be practiced at the wall or elevated with blocks. This stabilizing hip opener can open the root (muladhara) chakra. The opposing extension that occurs from tailbone to crown can rouse the crown (sahasrara) chakra. Because the abdominal wall is engaged to sustain the shape, the sacral (svadhisthana) chakra is activated.

THIS WEEK: WEIGH THE GOOD AND BAD

Whenever we're faced with a difficult decision, it can be tempting to seek counsel from others. Considering too many opinions in a choice that ought to be made by our own accord, however, can lead to more indecisiveness than when we first began our deliberations. With Libra energy abounding—always weighing the advantages and disadvantages to any situation—there is a tendency during this season to slip into the trap of analysis paralysis and avoid decision making entirely.

Reflect on a decision you currently face in your life: a lifestyle change, a move to another place, a job upgrade, or cutting ties with a toxic relationship. In your journal, create a good old-fashioned pros and cons list, bearing equal weight to each as best you can. Seeing on paper the frazzled thoughts that have been cycling through your mind may suddenly illuminate what it is you need to do to change course. This process will also remind you that whatever your circumstance, good or bad, eventually it too will pass.

DHARMA TALK

Our outer world
reflects our inner world,
a looking glass
that mirrors sensation
as the wheel of life spins round.
It is at the center of the cyclone
where harmony and stillness reside.
This galactic center
is our connection to the divine,
a balancing of yin and yang,
feminine and masculine,
good and bad,
light and dark—
a yoking of reality
in transcendence from
duality.

ABUNDANCE

Celebrating the Wholeness Within

Abundance is conflated with the external world: a full cornucopia of harvest, a bulging wallet, sufficient material possessions. The uneven distribution of resources in society creates an idea of scarcity. We are all in seeming competition for diminishing assets, and the global economy supports the stratification of "have" and "have not." But we are abundant, whole beings, integrally interconnected and complete. Scarcity is an illusion; we already have everything we need within.

Patanjali discusses abundance through two different lenses in the *Yoga Sutras.* The first is asteya, the third yama that directs us not to steal; the second is aparigraha, the fifth yama that directs us not to covet. Asteya teaches us that once the principle of non-stealing has been established, we enter a state of mental prosperity. By recognizing that we need not take from others, we define our sense of abundance. Aparigraha teaches the practice of non-attachment. When we release ourselves from comparison, we are able to see the depth of our inner well. Looking to others as a benchmark for our personal satisfaction or success creates the misconception of scarcity.

A yoga practice fosters feelings of wholeness. These glimpses of totality beget satisfaction with what we have versus what we do not. Lakshmi, the Hindu goddess of abundance and prosperity, is depicted as having four arms. Each of these represents one of the four basic principles of balanced, abundant living: moksha (liberation through connection to the divine), dharma (the act of right living), artha (material abundance), and kama (passion or enjoyment). When a person has experienced wholeness through these means, they live in Lakshmi's state of abundance.

Libra season and the start of autumn signify the waning harvest in preparation for the coming winter. Though the fields have been cleared, autumn is both an opportunity to take stock of abundance and make provision for the scarce winter months ahead. This polarity is a Libran theme, the zodiac sign that represents duality and is symbolized by Scales. Ruled by Venus, Libra attunes us to our heart center, reminding us to have compassion toward all living things.

PRACTICE

Bound Side Angle Pose
(Baddha Utthita Parsvakonasana)

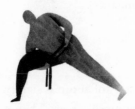

This expression of Side Angle Pose incorporates a bind to invite rotation of the torso by way of the rib cage to open the lungs, chest, and shoulders. A powerful, grounding standing twist, Bound Side Angle stretches and strengthens the ankles, quadriceps, glutes, and pelvic floor, mobilizes the thoracic spine, and stabilizes the abdominal wall. Rather than torquing your spine and forcing over-rotation, gently turn the rib cage to invite a natural rotation of your torso. A sense of anchoring is established by way of the outer edge of your back foot to help distribute weight evenly between both legs.

Work toward the bind by placing one hand to rest palm face-up at your lower back. Alternatively, both hands could reach for a piece of clothing or a strap placed between them.

A heart opener, Bound Side Angle stimulates the heart (anahata) chakra. With the feet pressing firmly to the ground, the root (muladhara) chakra is activated. Anchoring into our own foundation thwarts any temptation to compare ourselves to others. The fullness experienced in this shape allows us to be expansive in our external relationships and recognize our shared sense of abundance.

THIS WEEK: HARVEST MOON DINNER PARTY

Mabon is the pagan mid-harvest festival, traditionally celebrated on or near the equinox to give thanks for the bounty of the earth, while looking toward the coming winter. The harvest moon is always the first full moon of autumn, when crop yield is at its peak. Host a gathering with your family and friends on or near the harvest moon, and encourage everyone to bring a dish as a nod to shared abundance. Invoke the dharma arm of Lakshmi by sharing affirmations of gratitude before the meal; call upon kama by savoring each bite, eating slowly and intentionally. Make it a point to be gracious and complimentary to all your guests (practicing aparigraha), and to serve others at the table first (practicing asteya).

DHARMA TALK

You are enough, exactly as you are,
exactly as you were,
exactly as you will be.
You are an integral part of the
great gossamer of the divine,
of those you love, of those you've never met.
Connected as you are, how could
you ever be less?
The abundance of your wholeness proves the
illusion of scarcity, the delusion of paucity.
You have what you seek within.
You are everything you need.

TOLERANCE

Embodying Justice and Spreading Equality

If patience is a virtue, then tolerance—acceptance of ourselves and of each other—is divine. The five yamas in Patanjali's *Yoga Sutras* are described as tools of self-restraint and regulation. The first yama, ahimsa, teaches non-harming, or nonviolence. At its core, ahimsa is to renounce anger and hostility; practice of ahimsa can be taken to extremes through veganism or rejection of war. Yet ahimsa is not avoidance. It is to let others be as they are, despite differences. To harbor negative thoughts about others only cripples our capacity to live with ease.

When we realize we are spiritual beings having an experience in a body for a brief moment in time, we can more readily step into another person's shoes. When we objectively examine the vantage point of another, we are more capable of empathy. Acceptance of others as they are—without unfair judgment or unreasonable expectations—invites us to love and respect ourselves. The basic translation of "namaste" from Sanskrit is "the light in me honors the light in you," imploring us to bear witness to the very oneness and interconnectedness of all things, to realize that the other is also, in a sense, you.

This does not mean, however, that there is evil in the world that ought to be tolerated. To practice acceptance is to walk a fine line between intolerance of injustices and tolerance of the circumstances of our world—no matter how tumultuous those may be.

To rise above the duality of right and wrong, good and evil, we can look to the qualities of air sign Libra, symbolized by the Scales of Justice. The zodiac's peacekeeper, Libra has a reputation for being unable to take a stand. But there is power in impartiality, as both sides of the spectrum are carefully weighed. This theme presents itself during the fall season, when an election day looms and dichotomic issues can flare up. While tolerance is a component for peace, for outer harmony to be reached, some level of intolerance toward social injustices is necessary. It is our responses to those injustices that determine our inner equilibrium, however. We can still fight the good fight—but as peaceful warriors, as bearers of light.

PRACTICE

Scale Pose
(Tolasana)

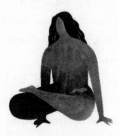

Scale Pose summons strength and stability of mind and body as an equalizer of effort and ease, as an embodiment of the Scales. This pose strengthens the shoulders and tones the arms while engaging the abdominals. It also increases flexibility in the hips while improving wrist flexion. By tilting the pelvis forward (spinal extension), you can rock the pelvis back (spinal flexion) and push the floor away with your hands to press up and float the legs.

If you have limited range of motion in the knee joints, trying this pose is not recommended. Instead, come to a kneeling posture (Thunderbolt, or Vajrasana), place hands on blocks to press down, and lift the weight of the knees and shins.

The root (muladhara) chakra opens as the pelvic floor muscles are activated. The core is engaged to stimulate the sacral (svadhisthana) and solar plexus (manipura) chakras. As the chest expands and the back body broadens, the heart (anahata) chakra is opened.

THIS WEEK: ORGANIZE A JUSTICE CIRCLE

These days, every year is an important election year. Assemble a justice league of like-minded humans to share knowledge and discuss political and social issues as a community. You might engage in mindful, nonargumentative dialogue—over some snacks and maybe even a drink or two—about various candidates on the local and national ballot, so that you're fully informed to cast your vote in a conscious and intentional manner.

Discuss the issues you care about, and practice tolerance when your opinions are challenged. With Libra being the sign of relationships, you could find that connecting with others in this way strengthens your bond and infuses your usual conversations with more substance and heart.

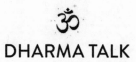

DHARMA TALK

When we are undivided,
interconnected and united,
we stand up for what is right,
we know when we must fight.
As harbingers of peace
we release false ideals
that fuel the fires of judgment.
When we tolerate each other
we cannot avoid or ignore
prejudice, famine,
and war after war.
If Lady Justice is blind,
our hands are not tied.
By spreading love and equality,
We become one with the divine.

LOVING-KINDNESS

Cultivating Warm-Hearted Feelings

Imagine a world where every person radiates kindness, compassion, and patience for one another, in which jealousy, spite, and frustration do not exist. This is the path of bhakti, one of the four main ancient yogic paths, alongside jñāna, raja, and karma. Bhakti yoga, Sanskrit for "devotion," teaches that liberation is found through connection to the divine, achieved by surrendering to the universal blissful love we innately possess.

There are nine steps of bhakti, beginning with the recognition of truth and reliance on faith. Next steps circumscribe practice and devotion, traditionally to a teacher. When we practice loving-kindness to ourselves, we can then share it outwardly with all beings. The result is an awakening of divine love within.

In the Buddhist tradition, the practice of loving-kindness is known as metta. Metta is one of the four sublime states put forth by Theravada Buddhism, along with compassion, equanimity, and empathetic joy. These attributes are also known as the four immeasurables, the successful employment of which leads to a Brahma state, a union with god consciousness.

Metta meditation, or metta bhavana, shares a similar foundational wisdom with the Hindu tradition: we are all one. As opposed to vipassana meditation, a style of sitting that cultivates personal insight, metta bhavana requires concentration. By first focusing loving-kindness inward, we develop the empathy necessary to then consciously direct that kindness, compassion, and patience outward. In so doing, we are working to become one with the divine.

Themes of love and romance are associated with Libra, the sign of partnerships and balance. By developing metta during Libra season, we hone the harmonious qualities this sign represents. Libra is an air sign that, despite projections of independence, can be reliant on others. Practicing loving-kindness reminds us that we are not alone in this world and that we are interdependent and interconnected.

PRACTICE

Camel Pose
(Ustrasana)

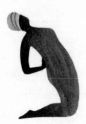

Camel Pose is named for the shape the body creates to resemble the hump of a camel's back. This heart-opening posture broadens the chest. The backbend does not come from pushing the pelvis forward but rather from spinal extension that begins in the lower back as the chest lifts.

Hands are placed on the lumbar for stability and support, as the crown of the head reaches back to maintain length in the cervical spine and stimulate the throat and thyroid. Bringing the tongue to the roof of your mouth can help keep the throat from constricting as the breath cycles in and out through your nose. You have the option to reach for your heels, though it's not necessary. To exit the pose safely, it is helpful to lead and lift with the heart, engaging the glutes and abdominals rather than pushing the hips forward.

Camel Pose ignites the heart (anahata) chakra to cultivate loving feelings of acceptance and compassion. The opening of the throat (vishuddha) chakra helps us to outwardly share these intentions of loving-kindness.

THIS WEEK: METTA MEDITATION

There is no better way to cultivate loving-kindness than a metta meditation practice. Begin in a comfortable seat, and choose affirming phrases that focus inward, such as, *May I be healthy. May I be safe. May I be free from suffering. May I be loved.* Concentrate on the feelings of warmth generated by the affirmations.

Next, bring to mind someone who loves you—a parent, a spouse, perhaps even a teacher. Imagine that person radiating their love to you, wishing that you be healthy, safe, free from suffering, and loved. Breathe deeply, and accept these feelings.

Next, send the same blessings to another person, perhaps someone with whom you have difficulty. You might try: *May you be healthy and safe. May you be free from suffering. May you be loved.* You can even send that blessing to a stranger, maybe someone you see on your morning commute or the person who brewed your latte.

When you're ready, begin to expand the blessings to all beings: *Just as I wish to be, may all beings be healthy, safe, and free. Just as I wish to be, may all beings be loved.*

Take note of how compassion and empathy begin to show up in other areas of your life.

DHARMA TALK

Kindness is more than gestures or gifts.
It is the recognition of small moments
as opportunities for greatness:
to smile at a stranger,
to give up your bus seat,
to help with a bag.
But we cannot give to the world
what we do not manifest within,
so hold close your kindness,
and let go of your fears.
You are of great value.
You are needed,
you are kind,
and you are love.

MANIFESTATION

You Are What You Attract

When was the last time you watched for "the signs"?

As the spiritual teacher Marianne Williamson (2014) posits in her book, *The Law of Divine Compensation,* manifestations are "miracles" that can happen when we shift our mindset. When we align with love and separate from fear, the universe conspires with us to help us realize our dreams and lead a life of prosperity. Changing your thoughts just might change your life.

The law of attraction claims that our thoughts have the power to create our reality. Those thoughts may present themselves as "coincidences," as the universe sends us signals to let us know we're on track. When Albert Einstein suggested that the most important question we can ask ourselves is whether the universe is a friendly or unfriendly place, he may have had this in mind. By believing that life is on our side, Einstein (n.d.) explained, we can explore the motives behind creation, learning how to work with the universe rather than against it.

While the law of attraction has not been proven by science, the Nobel Prize winner Max Planck, a collaborator of Einstein and the father of quantum mechanics, is said to have shared a similar belief. In an interview with *The Observer* in 1931, he noted that he regarded all matter as derived from consciousness (Schwartz 2018). Another Nobel Prize winner and physicist, Wolfgang Pauli, was an early explorer of quantum metaphysics and collaborated with the psychiatrist Carl Jung to study synchronicity, a term coined by Jung himself (Borowski 2012).

As science speculates, we can look to ancient texts to understand manifestation as a spiritual concept. In chapter 10 of the Bhagavad Gita (Easwaran 2007), "The Opulence of the Absolute," physical and spiritual manifestations of the universe are described as gifts from the Hindu deity Krishna, a supreme god. As Krishna revealed to Arjuna, the young hero and spiritual seeker of the story, when a yogi acknowledges the supreme powers of manifestation, they are connected to the divine, which, in turn, invites the divine to work with and through them.

The focus to manifest our visions falls into the intensity of Scorpio's domain. Ruled by Pluto, Scorpionic energy is powerful, transformative, even karmic. Scorpio governs our long-term finances and material resources, as well as how we share our power and wealth. As the current calendar year begins to wind down, during Scorpio season we may find ourselves beginning to visualize some of our bigger-picture goals.

PRACTICE

Sphinx Pose
(Salamba Bhujangasana)

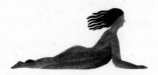

Since Ancient Egyptian times, the mythical sphinx has served as a symbol of mystery, fascination, and intrigue. This heart-opening posture embodies the lower, grounded phase of Scorpionic energy and invites a laser focus, or drishti, from a place of ease. Sphinx Pose stretches the abdominal muscles while strengthening the glutes. By rooting into the forearms, the thoracic spine is mobilized. Pressing into the tops of your feet, pubis, and thigh bones can mitigate strain in the lumbar, and a slight engagement of the glutes helps protect that region.

As the top of your head extends upward to open your crown (sahasrara) chakra, you can think of this as an energetic exchange between the underworld below and the heavens above. The throat (vishuddha) chakra is also opened as you extend your cervical spine. As your internal gaze is brought to the third-eye (ajna) chakra, your intuition and powers of visualization become heightened.

THIS WEEK: VISION BOARD DREAM CRAFTING

Olympic athletes use visualization techniques when competing, and neuroscientific studies have proven its effectiveness (Loder 2014). Create a vision board to physically identify what it is you seek, crafting an intuitive road map to get there. If the law of attraction states that whatever can be imagined by the mind can be achieved, why not put those visions into material form as a daily reminder of what you intend to make manifest?

Vision boarding can be done by yourself or with a friend or a group. Grab a stack of magazines, photographs, scissors, and glue. Choose images that inspire you and are in alignment with your goals—that is, whatever you wish to magnetize into your life. You might cut out phrases or letters to string together your own affirmations or mantras too—especially if you have limiting beliefs surrounding money, work, or your abilities. There is no wrong way to make a vision board, so long as you're giving yourself permission to express your dreams in physical form.

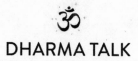

DHARMA TALK

We are cocreators
with the cosmos,
wise as the skies,
old as stardust.
When we trust
what we believe
we are able to receive
all that is coming
and all that we need.

32

INTENSITY

Savoring the Details of Experience

It is in the smallest of details where we can plug into the intensity of an experience. The tiniest drops of hail herald the strength of an autumn storm; the deep red and orange hues of metamorphosing leaves generate the fiery blaze of a fall landscape. Tuning into the simplicity of body-breath connection allows us to tap into the fervency of practice. As we cultivate sensation through movement and observation, we are able to savor the clarity of the here and now.

The flow state is a state of consciousness coined by the Hungarian-American psychologist Mihaly Csikszentmihalyi and is described as an experience of total immersion in the moment. Also referred to as "being in the flow," this energized focus propagates a greater appreciation for whatever the task at hand may be. Flow states are breeding grounds for lasting joy, contentment, and satisfaction.

Rasa, a concept in Hindu philosophy, loosely translates to "the particular quality, or essence, of an artistic pursuit" such as dance or theater. First outlined in the *Natyashastra,* a handbook of dramatic art for traditional Sanskrit theater, the rasa theory calls for performance to be not only entertaining but transformative. The audience should be transported into the story so fully that they are able to subconsciously explore deep moral and spiritual themes.

Though not traditionally associated with asana, rasa theory encourages us to work toward mind-body transformation, to enter a flow state beyond the physical realm.

Intensity is a Scorpionic theme. People born under this sun sign are associated with almost inhuman laser focus, an ability to delve into whatever task or experience is at hand with absolute attention. During Scorpio season, we may feel compelled to devote ourselves entirely to one particular project or goal, or investigate a recurring behavior or pattern in our lives. Symbolized by the Scorpion, Scorpio rules the reproductive system and sex organs, the sacral center of our energetic body. With Pluto, the god of the underworld, as Scorpio's cosmic guardian, themes of transformation arise. We may experience intense emotional and physical connections from the sacral center, as well as in our relationships to ourselves and with others.

PRACTICE

Pyramid Pose
(Parsvottanasana)

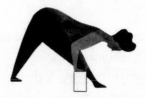

Pyramid Pose, also known as Intense Side Stretch Pose, is an inversion that offers an intense stretch along the hips, hamstrings, and shoulders. Plugging into the outer edges of the feet invites a slight external rotation of the thighs to stabilize the SI hip joints so that the pelvis can remain more or less neutral. Allowing the knees to bend and soften can relax the lumbar and facilitate a neutral spine as you hinge forward. Pyramid Pose can improve balance and core strength, as well as strengthen the legs.

Place your hands on blocks to elevate the shape for more accessibility, or keep your back heel lifted. You can also flip your palms and point your fingertips backward to stretch your wrists and triceps. If there is enough stability in your pelvis and core, bring your hands behind your back into a reverse prayer to open your chest.

This stretch encourages the flow of apana, downward- or outward-moving breath. Folding forward at the pelvis stimulates the flow of energy from the solar plexus (manipura) and sacral (svadhisthana) chakras—particularly through the back body. Anchoring the feet into the earth bolsters the root (muladhara) chakra.

THIS WEEK: FREEWRITE IN THE FLOW

Freewriting can be done daily without a specific intent or ritualized to achieve a certain outcome or goal. Wake up ten minutes earlier than you normally would and journal in a favorite, solitary spot in your home. Or begin writing while still in bed, before the subconscious meanderings of your mind yield to the more pressing matters of the day. Allow your thoughts to pour onto paper without worrying that they make sense, work together, or even lead to a conclusion. Try this every day for at least a week. Notice how quickly you're able to immerse into the flow state. And be sure to look back and read what you wrote to self-evaluate what helps get you there.

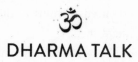

DHARMA TALK

The surrender of self to the flow of the mind—
the release of the physical world
to the transformative
engagement of experience—
this is how we swim with
the currents of conscious existence,
how we sail upon the waters
of our singular here and now.

33

UNRAVELING

Learning to Accept Transition

As leaves start to change and the air begins to chill, we've shed the levity of summer as we prepare for hibernation and anticipate the release of winter. What happens in between is the unraveling of the ego, the letting go of our need to control, the yoking of body and breath as presence is reestablished.

In sankhya philosophy—one of the six Hindu schools of thought—the world is perceived as existing of two opposing realities: prakriti (tangible matter) and purusha (consciousness). In practice, we learn to release ourselves from the bondage of prakriti and move into the stream of purusha. We begin to untangle the trappings of ego and expectation, known in Vedic context as ahamkara. In the Bhagavad Gita, Krishna directs Arjuna to release himself from the state of prakriti, as the true self (existing in the state of purusha) can never be present when shackled by ahamkara.

The unraveling of the ego and the resulting connection to purusha are some of the heart's greatest and most challenging work. Autumn, of course, is an apt time to explore this idea of transition; yet it's not seasonally exclusive. Life is cyclical. We will wind up and bind to the ego—and then unravel, release, and grow again and again.

Like a phoenix rising from the ashes or a serpent shedding its skin, unraveling invokes the qualities of Scorpio. As the Scorpion, this sign is associated with destruction and samsara, the cycle of life, death, and rebirth. Ruled by Pluto, the planet of transformation, Scorpionic energy may drive us to unbind ourselves from false patterns. The end goal, of course, is not to eradicate the self but to refine—and maybe even find some form of salvation. Scorpio's energy encourages us to become the phoenix, to continue the journey onward and upward, and to continually seek the unraveling of that which may keep us from truly knowing ourselves.

PRACTICE

Eagle Pose
(Garudasana)

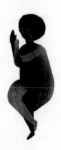

Eagle Pose is named for Garuda, the mythical king of the birds, portrayed as having an eagle's beak, an impressive bright red wingspan, and the golden body of a man. According to the Mahabharata, Garuda's mother, Vinata, mother of the birds, was tricked into becoming a slave to her sister-wife, mother of the serpents. The serpents agreed to release her from servitude if Garuda could bring them the elixir of immortality—which he did, giving snakes the ability to shed their skin and be born anew.

Eagle Pose can be modified depending on range of motion. In lieu of a wrap, you may actively press forearms and palms together and lift elbows to shoulder height as the shoulder blades protract apart. Wrapping the legs generates sensation in the IT band, which connects the hip to the knee, but does not lengthen the same way that muscles do. You can invite more stability into the shape by pressing the top of the wrapped foot into the back of the opposite calf muscle or by balancing the big toe on the ground. It is not necessary to fold forward. Draw the torso slightly back in space to remain upright.

Eagle Pose is a standing pose that activates the root (muladhara) chakra. The core engages to maintain the balance, awakening the solar plexus (manipura) chakra. As with any balancing pose, Eagle Pose is sustained with a drishti, a point of soft, concentrated focus. This stimulates the third-eye (ajna) chakra. The upward flow of energy from the traditional, familial center to one's personal power center and toward the center of intuition is an empowering sensation.

THIS WEEK: FULL MOON MUSINGS

The full moon is a potent time of transition, a time to release the ego with an intention of phoenix-like transformation and growth. This full moon ritual can be done alone or in a circle of people you trust. Grab two sheets of paper. Divide the top sheet into two columns: in the first, write down what you're ready to release, what you're willing to unravel. Copy the first column into the second, and tear off the second column, one statement at a time. Recite each one to yourself, and then—carefully—light them on fire and extinguish them in a bowl of water. When you've finished, use the other sheet to write next to the first column how you will transform from that which you've released.

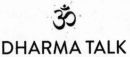

DHARMA TALK

Just as the moon waxes and wanes
from brightness to darkest night,
so too do we perpetually
unravel, rebuild, set ablaze, rethread.
There is death in life—there is no way around it.
But there too is life in death.
And so we go forward, beat onward,
releasing into darkness and rebuilding into light,
every season, every practice, every life.

34

REBIRTH

Rising from the Ashes

Ephemeral seasons are paradoxical in nature: autumn connects the warmth of summer with the frigidity of winter. It is a time to acknowledge the culmination of harvest and prepare for the coming exiguity. The transitory phase of fall asks us to carefully consider that which is enriching our lives and that which no longer serves us.

Throughout ancient cosmogonies, deities reflect a similar duality—Kali, for example, is the Hindu goddess of destruction and rebirth. Often depicted wearing a necklace of skulls or standing on Shiva's prostrate body, Kali is the destroyer of the ego and the liberator of souls. Her name comes from the Sanskrit word "kāla," which means "time," the immutable procession of nature that perpetuates samsara: the cycle of life, death, and rebirth.

Vaisheshika is one of the six orthodox schools of Hindu thought. In Vaisheshika philosophy, both time (kāla) and space are recognized as nonlinear, without beginning or end. The concept of kāla can be applied in a number of ways, one of which measures the phases of the moon. There are approximately fifteen nights during each waxing and waning period—fifteen nights from the full moon to a new moon. The idea of the sixteenth kāla reminds us of a Kali-like dyadic of destruction and rebirth: even under the darkness of a new moon, though we cannot see it, we trust that the light is there. Only when we have faced the darkest of nights can we walk into the brilliance of dawn.

Rebirth is a Scorpio theme, as this sign is ruled by Pluto, the planet of death and transformation. The self-destruction often associated with Scorpionic energy isn't spurred by a desire to simply immolate, however, but to rise from the ashes, a phoenix transformed by the salvation of shedding and transition. A water sign associated with the reproductive center, Scorpio comprises four personifications: the venomous scorpion, the cunning but seductive snake, the hawkish eagle able to circle its prey, and the phoenix, emerging victorious from the flame. Each is an integral stage in the cycle of destruction to rebirth, of darkness to light.

PRACTICE

Dancer's Pose
(Natarajasana)

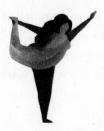

Natarajasana is named for the depiction of Shiva Nataraja, king of the dance. This is the incantation of Shiva, whose furious, destructive dance propels forth the cycle of life—immortalizing Shiva as creator, preserver, and destroyer. Shiva Nataraja is shown stepping on Apasmara, a soul bound by ignorance and earthly pursuit.

Dancer's Pose is a heart and chest opener that mobilizes the shoulder girdle and stretches the upper body as well as the thighs and groins. A stable footing is essential for maintaining balance. To avoid compression in your lower back, send your pelvis slightly back in space and focus on lifting the thigh rather than kicking the foot into the hand.

As you hinge forward, keep your chest lifted to open the heart (anahata) chakra. The sacral (svadhisthana) and solar plexus (manipura) chakras also become activated. When moving through the cycle of samsara, we must reexamine our deepest desires as well as what ignites our fire.

THIS WEEK: RELEASE THE EXCESS

We've all heard stories of a bad breakup situation, some of which may have resulted in the destruction of relationship memorabilia. But ridding yourself of that which no longer serves you does not always have to be an extreme gesture.

For one week, write down your daily schedule—to the hour. Be honest with yourself about what you're really doing with your time: if you're lying in bed scrolling through social media for fifteen minutes every morning, make note of it. Once you have this understanding of how you're spending your time, go through and take stock of that which helps you grow, learn, or develop; on the flipside note what doesn't. Re-create your schedule so that you fill your time with all of the things that bolster the best version of yourself.

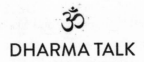

DHARMA TALK

Doing the work isn't done alone—
but it's part of the cycle of release and rebirth.
From great loss comes great growth;
in transition we begin to evolve.
Just as the phoenix must first face the flame,
so too do we endure the heat to
step into our truest selves.

GRATITUDE

Our Countless Blessings

It is easy to lose sight of the myriad gifts our lives have bestowed upon us. We become mired in in the ego, seeking status and recognition. The trappings of this focused self-importance hinder spiritual progress and convince us that we are not enough; the mind perpetuates an illusion that having "more" enhances self-worth. It is the nature of the mind to fixate on problems and lack, to cling to scarcity out of fear.

In the *Yoga Sutras,* Patanjali describes "non-grasping" to material things as aparigraha. When we recognize the abundance of all that we have and all we are able to do, we enrich our perspectives. From this place of perceived bounty we are able to evolve and ascend. Recognizing that true opulence is within cultivates deeper satisfaction and lasting fulfillment, and infuses our lives with meaning.

At the intersection of spirituality and science is the field of positive psychology, which posits that a positive attitude of gratitude is key to mental and physical well-being. Robert Emmons, a professor of psychology at the University of California, Davis, is renowned for his research on the benefits a gratitude practice can have on health and happiness. Emmons (2010) has described this mindset as a "chosen attitude": when we are consciously grateful for what we have versus what we do not, we have actively made a choice to be happy.

Imagine what might transpire if the developed world could acknowledge that free will determines the degree to which we experience happiness.

In the United States, Thanksgiving arrives alongside the start of Sagittarius season. Despite the problematic historical context of the holiday, it is nevertheless an occasion to celebrate our bountiful gifts with loved ones. Sagittarius is the ninth sign of the zodiac, symbolized by the wise Archer. Ruled by Jupiter, the largest body in our solar system and the mythical god of feast, the Archer reminds us of all that is possible—but not without adopting the high-minded rectitude of being grateful for what we have first. Karmically, we cannot expect the universe to reciprocate and make manifest our visions when we do not honor its blessings.

PRACTICE

Garland Pose
(Malasana)

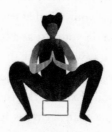

Sagittarius rules the hips, and this squatting posture is known for its capacity to strengthen the pelvic floor. As the hip flexors and groins receive a deep stretch, the shape also strengthens the ankles and feet. The abdominal wall engages slightly to activate the posterior chain and to maintain a neutral spine and upright torso. Garland Pose, also known as Squat Pose, can be made more accessible by placing a block beneath the seat for support. This helps to build stability in the ankle joints and root into the outer edges of the feet.

Draw your palms together at your heart as a gesture of gratitude. Press your elbows into the lowest part of your inner thighs to facilitate hip opening. Alternatively, the inner edges of your feet can be brought together to send the knees out wide as your spine rounds or flexes forward. This foundational pose engages the root (muladhara) chakra and stimulates the sacral (svadhisthana) chakra.

THIS WEEK: WRITE THANK-YOU NOTES

It is beneficial to keep a gratitude journal and carve out time each day to reflect on your many blessings, regardless of their significance. Freewriting about what you're thankful for in the morning helps set the tone for the rest of your day. Reflecting on what you're grateful for at the end of each day puts your mind at ease, especially when you're able to consider each item on your list as a beautiful gift.

Think of this practice as writing a thank-you note to your higher self. You could even choose to hone your focus on a specific entity in your life—maybe a person. Explore the thoughts and feelings that arise when you realize the many reasons for your gratitude as you write them down. Notice the richness you feel each time you perform the exercise. Bonus activity: send someone a handwritten thank-you note that expresses your admiration and appreciation.

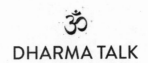

DHARMA TALK

Every day is a gift—
an opportunity to breathe, to smile, to be kind.
Though it is easy to forget,
we are here to remember
just how beautiful it is to be alive.
To be truly thankful, to count our blessings
is to commune with the self,
to converse with the divine.

36

EXPANSION

The Precipice of Possibility

Yoga is a practice of expansion, a broadening of body that creates spaciousness in the mind as the scope of perception widens. The practice of presence reveals how to release limiting beliefs and expectations, how to broaden our horizons and transform our realities. This process of changing our circumstances requires stepping outside of our comfort zones. To take a bold leap of faith is to accept the possibility of failure. By navigating that which is necessary for our continued development, we hone our unique purpose in this life.

As we attain milestones, we will inevitably reach a point when we ask ourselves, *What's next?* Expansion isn't a destination but a journey. Our successes are maps for the next road to take. In the Tao Te Ching, Laozi writes that the farther you travel, the less you know (Ames and Hall, 2004). Each new door that is opened leads us to experiences we didn't even know we could have. To expand is to empower ourselves to traverse the unknown.

Exploring your edge is an examination of boundaries and self-imposed limitations. If you've reached a plateau in your practice, it's worth considering where in your life this same standstill might be mirrored. By drawing from the fiery source of spirit, we expand the ways in which we see ourselves and the world around us, and rekindle the flame of our ambitions. This is the difference between a fixed mindset and a growth mindset: when we believe that the only limits we face are the ones we put on ourselves, we are expanding our perception.

The fearless enthusiasm of fire sign Sagittarius inspires us to explore what is possible. Sagittarius is a visionary, ruled by Jupiter, the planet of good fortune that reminds us that stagnancy only keeps us small. Symbolized by the courageous Archer, Sagittarius encourages us to take a chance—a reminder that risk yields reward. As we stand at the precipice of possibility and plunge forth into the unknown, the excitement of taking a gamble in the game of life broadens our perspectives, regardless of outcome.

PRACTICE

Warrior III
(Virabhadrasana III) with Jupiter Mudra

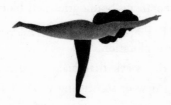

Hindu mythology describes the warrior Virabhadra, an incarnation of Shiva, in three aspects, providing fodder for all three Warrior poses. When Daksha, a powerful priest, did not invite his daughter Sati or her husband, Shiva, to a ritual sacrifice, Sati threw herself in the fire in retaliation. Sometimes called Balancing Stick Pose, Warrior III's shape comes from the moment in the story when Virabhadra (Shiva) offers Daksha's decapitated head forward. (See Warrior II, page 65, for an extended story.)

Warrior III stabilizes the hips and strengthens the back body and the abdominal wall. The shape tests and improves balance, and requires total-body coordination. Jupiter mudra can be incorporated into the pose by interlocking the palms overhead and extending the index fingers toward one's expansiveness, to the vast possibilities of the future.

The throat (vishuddha) chakra is activated by both the posture and the mudra as the cervical spine extends. The crown (sahasrara) chakra awakens to the higher collective consciousness, and the third-eye (ajna) chakra is roused to greater insight and clarity. The sacral (svadhisthana) and solar plexus (manipura) chakras are also stimulated.

THIS WEEK: TRY SOMETHING THAT SCARES YOU

A world of possibility becomes available when we recognize the privilege of choice. So why is it we are so quick to place finite expectations on ourselves? To demarcate boundaries and blockades, rather than recognize the infinite possibilities available to us? The potentialities of the world beg for exploration.

Do one thing this week that makes you uncomfortable. This could be something new or something you've tried before but then shied away from. Your mission is to navigate discomfort from a place of ease. This could be anything from a truth-telling social media post to trying a group fitness class or even bungee jumping. The possibilities for this are limitless. Like Bruce Lee said, "There are no limits, only plateaus." You may also benefit from writing about this experience in your journal.

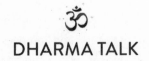

DHARMA TALK

Just as the vast cosmos are infinite,
so too is universal potential.
To settle is to hinder freedom and liberation,
to expand is to rewrite beliefs
of what we think is possible.
When we recognize each moment
as limitless potential,
we become expansive
in our wholeness.

37

BRAVERY

Moving Through Fear into Courage

Courage does not always mean there is no fear. We will always be confronted with difficulty and duress that may plague us with anxiety and concern. It is how we choose to react and learn from these situations that builds our character and shapes our moral compass. It is not an act of courage to go on living when a loved one has died, for example, though it is brave to accept the loss and continue to build a life without them.

Parvati is the Hindu goddess of courage, often associated with the depiction of a lion or the deity Nandi (the gatekeeper to Shiva's home) and the symbol of the crossbow. She is also the incarnation of the divine mother, Adi Parashakti, or Adishakti. Calling upon the divine mother, the primary creative power, invokes the courage to move through insecurities and into one's personal power.

To overcome feelings of insecurity is to release ourselves from fear, to deny self-perpetuated sentiments that we aren't enough. To embrace our personal power is an act of bravery. It takes courage to accept oneself fully, to accept that we are deserving of that which we seek.

Sagittarius is symbolized by the brave Archer with a bow and arrow. It is during Sagittarius season when we may consider personal and professional risks as we look toward another year's end—when perhaps we have nothing to lose. In Greek mythology, the constellation Sagittarius is associated with Chiron, the centaur who taught Achilles the archery skills that would lead him to notoriety in the Trojan War.

Sagittarius is ruled by Jupiter, the planet of expansion, optimism, and growth. This energy encourages us to stretch our horizons through exploration, travel, and learning. Exploration requires courage from the seeker: we cannot expand until we fearlessly confront the limitations we have placed on ourselves.

PRACTICE

Bow Pose
(Dhanurasana)

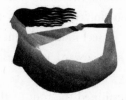

The seven-hundred-verse conversation in the Bhagavad Gita between Krishna and Arjuna occurs when Arjuna puts down his dhanu (weapon-bow) and refuses to fight. Krishna works to convince Arjuna that the battle is in fact his dharma and part of the greater plan. The bow shape of this posture is an archetype for cultivating courage in the face of transition, to surrender the ego and go forth with fearlessness and grace.

Bow Pose is a tremendous backbend. Though the shape asks the hip flexors to move beyond a functional range of motion, you can make Bow Pose more accessible by using a strap. As your back body is activated and abdominals receive a stretch, Bow Pose broadens your chest and pectoral muscles across the front of your body to open your heart. Extension is generated from tailbone to crown, particularly along the cervical spine, to open your throat.

This posture is energetically significant, as the heart (anahata) chakra is the point of transition from the lower (material) chakras, and the upper (spiritual) energetic centers. Bow Pose also activates the throat (vishuddha) chakra, stimulating courage to voice our authentic truths.

THIS WEEK: ACKNOWLEDGE YOUR FEARS

Write down three things that scare you. These can be weighty concepts—death, being alone, and so forth—or everyday occurrences, such as taking an elevator or getting lost. Then spend some time examining why it is you think this thing scares you. Are you afraid of being alone because you don't think you'll be able to survive? Or because you don't want to feel lonely? Acknowledging the source of your fears is the first step toward laying the framework to move through them.

Once you have determined the root of these fears, define small ways to address it. If you're afraid of being alone, try turning off your phone and spend a full day without relying on anyone else to show you that you'll be okay. If you're afraid of taking an elevator, try taking it just one floor up. When we give credence to our fears and remind ourselves that even what scares us most is changeable, we create a pathway for courage.

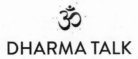

DHARMA TALK

It is not courageous to be without fear
but to acknowledge and release oneself from it.
Fear is not immutable but a pathway that
requires us to walk toward our truest self.
When we face the darkness of fear,
we step into the bravery of light.
You have the courage within
to become the warrior you seek.

AUTHENTICITY

Discovering and Loving
Who You Are

The concept of authenticity gets thrown around often in our modern world. Groups varying from the hippies to the punk rockers to twentieth-century existentialists grappled with defining what it meant to be authentic. The hippies bucked the mainstream; the punk rockers defined "poseur." Sartre presented the idea of "facticity," concrete truths inherent to all living beings, positing that authenticity is immutable (Messerly 2014).

Satya is the second of the yamas, described by Patanjali in the *Yoga Sutras*. Known as "truthfulness," satya asks us to slow down, restrain our speech, and consider our words before speaking. This quiet reflection allows us to express ourselves more authentically. Satya is also meant to encourage ahimsa, or non-harming. Speaking truth is a step toward wise action and authentic wholeness, asking that we resist the urge to speak in such a way that could cause direct harm to another.

Satya relates to the niyama that instructs us to self-inspect: svadhyaya, which reveals our vulnerabilities—a crucial step on the journey toward authenticity. When we face the obstacles on our path with courage and honesty, we live from a place of truth. When we identify the areas in our lives that need to be strengthened—and take action to make those changes—we are stepping into our most authentic self.

Authenticity is inherently optimistic, because it requires the courage to speak truth. Optimism, after all, is the cornerstone of courage. Symbolized by the confident Archer, Sagittarius is the great optimist of the zodiac, both self-assured and self-possessed. Ruled by Jupiter, the auspicious planet of faith and luck, Sagittarius energy encourages the deep work of aspiring to one's highest self, of discovering our true authentic selves.

PRACTICE

Cat and Cow
(Marjaryasana and Bitilasana)

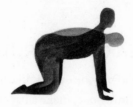

A practice of physical svadhyaya is a great way to begin an authentic conversation with your body. Cat and Cow invite you to explore intuitive movement. You can begin with side-to-side lateral flexion of the spine and even try circling the hips. From a neutral spine, try placing the hands just wide of the elbows, and knees just behind the hips, for more functionality, which can help facilitate spinal flexion and extension between the two postures. Press the floor away to lift the back of the heart and round your spine into Cat, and try not to collapse your shoulders as you broaden your chest to come into Cow. The Cat and Cow sequence mobilizes the thoracic spine and strengthens the shoulder girdle and back muscles. It also helps with stability in Sagittarius-ruled hips and creates spaciousness in the chest while toning the abdominal wall.

Both Cat and Cow work in conjunction to open the throat (vishuddha) and heart (anahata) chakras, as well as stimulate the sacral (svadhisthana) chakra, just below the navel, and the solar plexus (manipura) chakra, just above. Because the entirety of the spinal cord is working to facilitate these movement patterns, the root (muladhara) as well as the crown (sahasrara) chakras are also activated. Like a nourishing tonic for the chakra system, Cat and Cow, simple and basic as they may seem, are perhaps two of the most powerful shapes for unblocking and realigning all of the chakras.

THIS WEEK: SPEAK YOUR TRUTH

With a trusted friend who may be on a similar journey of self-discovery or interested in beginning one, make a list of the different areas of your lives you're looking to investigate. Sit down facing each other and try to maintain eye contact as you go through the list and take turns pronouncing at least one true statement for each topic. Your statements should be ones that, when spoken, help to illuminate a plan of action forward.

Dig deep and take your time. For example, if the item on the list is "Be respected at work," a potential truth could be: "I'm often scared to stand up for myself and seek acknowledgment for what I do." Working with a friend will also provide accountability for follow-through on your action plan, once you've each identified your truths.

DHARMA TALK

You are a unique being, the only you
who has ever breathed, moved, or loved.
Because you are the only one, how
could you not be the perfect expression of
your own singular humanity?
To be true to yourself is to
recognize the innate splendor of your being,
to honor the process of your becoming into
the immediate here and now.
You are perfect, real, and authentically
where you need to be.

WISDOM

Awakening the Guru Within

Is wisdom in the stars or found in books? Does it reside outside of ourselves or does it come from within? All wisdom originated somewhere—earned and shared by those who unraveled a discovery, a solution, an invention. But inner wisdom came from somewhere too. Be it a god or some other higher power, there is a spiritual intelligence that exists within the fabric of the universe—one that has been given many names since the dawn of humankind. This wisdom may present itself to us as a feeling, a tingle, or sensation—and it is, in all truthfulness, based in the belief that there is an unseen force driving all of creation.

Like knowledge, wisdom is powerful when we wield it. Knowledge, however, requires proof and reminds us that the more we know, the less we know. No great discoveries were made without first possessing an inner knowing or inkling—the answers to what we seek originate from within. Wisdom springs from the universal source that is always working with us and pulsating through us—available when we need it, teaching us grace, patience, ease, and contentment. This is an acknowledgment of the inner, knowing self and its unlimited potential.

We cannot understand or accept the world outside of us until we acknowledge our inner teacher. In sutra 1.26, Patanjali defines the ancient, timeless guru—the divine—as "the teacher of all teachers." If we look to the meaning of namaste and the very essence of yoga, we can acknowledge that within each and every one of us there is indeed a light: a teacher, a creator, guru, or god.

Wisdom invokes the archetype of the philosophical Archer representing Sagittarius, the zodiac's most perspective-broadening sign. Sagittarius energy is wise beyond its years. It invites us to illuminate the truth from an inherent, intuitive place in an effort to awaken the guru within. Ruled by Jupiter, the planet that rouses our most outspoken and worldly natures, Sagittarius's thirst for knowledge is never quite sated. The high-minded Archer also draws us toward the metaphysical realm in a seemingly unending quest for mind expansion and soul enrichment.

PRACTICE

Easy Seat
(Sukhasana)

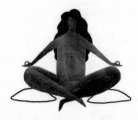

When Prince Siddhartha sat beneath the Bodhi tree for seven weeks to understand the meaning of existence, he vowed not to leave his seat until he could find a way to end the suffering of the world around him—even if that meant his own death. During those forty-nine days, he realized that the cause of human suffering was greed, selfishness, and foolishness, and that if we could rid ourselves of these senseless emotions we could find true happiness and contentment. With this revelation, he attained enlightenment and reemerged as the Buddha.

This simple seated posture helps relax and open the hips and groins—the region of the body ruled by Sagittarius—and lengthen the outer thigh muscles, or abductors, as well as stretch the ligaments in the knees and ankles. By holding the spine upright, the back muscles are strengthened. If the hips and knees are tight, sit on top of a folded blanket or a yoga block for additional support. In meditation, Easy Seat, or any comfortable seat, relieves stress and anxiety when attention is redirected to the breath.

Energetically, there is a sense of grounding into the sitting bones to activate the root (muladhara) chakra at the base of the spine.

The Yoga Almanac

Because the entire spine is being held upright, there is a lengthening from tailbone to crown that could essentially open all seven chakras.

THIS WEEK: SIT IN STILLNESS

As Socrates put it so eloquently: "As above, so below. As within, so without." We cannot know the outside world until we truly know ourselves. And we cannot truly know ourselves unless we look within and connect to source.

Set a timer for fifteen to twenty minutes and take a comfortable seat with your back supported. There's no need to force yourself into a "perfect posture" or seat; you have the option to change your position or even lie down at any point, if need be. For the duration of this seat recite the mantra "Wahe [wah-hay] guru" softly in your mind until it slowly fades into the background. If your mind starts to wander, pause, and then bring yourself back to the mantra.

This Kundalini mantra of wisdom invokes the teacher within. It translates loosely as, "I am in ecstasy when I experience the indescribable wisdom." Breathe deeply, observing the rise and fall of your belly with breath for the duration of your seat.

DHARMA TALK

What begins as a whisper,
wisdom begs to be heard.
And when that calling is ignored,
wisdom will show us the way—
whether we like it or not,
whether we're ready or not.
Like the metamorphosis
of chrysalis to mature butterfly,
wisdom is the force
behind all transformation.

WINTER

The Quiet Inward Journey

Capricorn ◉ Aquarius ◉ Pisces

"The quieter you become,
the more you are able to hear."

—Rumi

Winter marks the beginning of a new solar year as the Gregorian calendar nears its culmination, signifying the completion of another cycle before the reemergence of spring. For thousands of years, the winter solstice, the shortest day of the year, has been celebrated as a return to light, a return to innocence, an inevitable rebirth as the world continues to spin.

Also known as midwinter and the hibernal solstice, the solstice occurs around December 21 or 22 each year and marks the beginning of the winter season in the Northern Hemisphere. On the solstice, the sun appears at its lowest point in the sky, hovering directly over the Tropic of Capricorn.

This spiritual homecoming has metamorphosed into what we know in Christian tradition as Christmas on December 25. Long before that, the pagan festival Saturnalia had marked the start of winter, as did the birthday of the "invincible" sun god, Sol Invictus, during the golden age of the Roman Empire. In Ancient Egypt, January 6 was first recognized as winter's coming, which was later adopted by Christianity as the Feast of the Epiphany.

In Western astrology, this coincides with the start of Capricorn season, the most ambitious sign of the zodiac and synonymous with goal setting. During this cycle, we are invited to realign with our highest ideals as we look toward the year ahead—despite that we're in the throes of the holiday season.

Capricorn is symbolized by the unusual paradox that is the Sea Goat, a testament to the persistent energy of this ambitious yet grounded earth sign. Ruled by Saturn, the tough teacher planet known throughout astrological lore as Father Karma, Capricorn is also associated with the root (muladhara) chakra, reminding us that we must anchor our lofty dreams and grand visions in reality. Refining our intentions during Capricorn season can help us develop a blueprint for our plans, just in time for Aquarius season to begin (around January 20).

Aquarius is a radical, high-minded air sign that shifts our collective focus toward the future and a better planet, and is ruled by Uranus, the planet of innovation. In the Vedic tradition, the humanitarian Water Bearer was also governed by Saturn—long before Uranus was discovered. As Pisces season arrives (around February 19), we have reached the completion of the zodiac wheel and can work on healing, processing, and, ultimately, releasing. As the twelfth and final sign of the zodiac, symbolized by two Fish swimming in opposite directions, Pisces governs endings and closure. A water sign ruled by Neptune, god of the seas, Pisces is mystical and intuitive by nature.

Ayurveda describes winter as a kaphic season with underlying vata qualities. The slow-moving, heavy energy that winter brings sends many animals into hibernation and could steer yoga practitioners toward more introspective modalities such as yin, restorative, or meditation. Dry, crisp, and brisk qualities of later winter bring vata elements into play and may lead to feelings of isolation.

In Native American medicine wheel traditions, winter is associated with the elder wisdom of the North. The spirit keeper of the North is the buffalo or bison, an animal totem noted for its strength and resilience, power, and steadfastness. The quietness of the winter season gives us pause to reflect on the broader spectrum of life. It is in contemplative inquiry that we can view life from its deepest depths to highest heights and begin to understand that difficulty and ease can coexist. Winter is a reminder that we don't have to feel lonely when we're alone, that time spent in isolation can be nurturing. Only when we traverse through the darkness and find solace within the solitude of the season can we step forward into the light and become reborn again come spring.

40

INTENTION

The Starting Point of a Dream

An intention is a refinement of larger goals that we set for ourselves. In yogic tradition, a sankalpa is a resolution for determining your heart's desires. It comes from the Sanskrit root "san," which translates to "higher truth," and "kalpa," which means "vow or promise." When we have determined the heart's resolve, we can then philosophically align with the actions and goals that support it.

Though intentions can be set at any time of year, winter is a felicitous time to do so. We set intentions or resolutions for the new year to help hone our focus and consider where we need to correct course. Through refinement of our goals, the intentions we set help to steer us toward our highest potential.

It is common practice to set an intention at the beginning of a yoga class. How will that class direct your attention or help you move toward your sankalpa? With practice, the intentions we nurture will inevitably become part of our nature, amplifying who we are now and guiding us like a compass toward who we were born to be. As we peel back the layers of routine and witness the path ahead with clearer vision, we more readily align with our true calling.

The winter solstice coincides with the start of Capricorn season, the most goal-oriented phase of the zodiac that calls us to recalibrate our objectives. Capricorn is symbolized by the unusual paradox that is the Sea Goat, a testament to the persistent energy of this ambitious yet sturdy sign. Capricorn is ruled by Saturn, the tough teacher planet known in astrological lore as Father Karma. A grounded earth sign, Capricorn reminds us that lofty dreams and grand visions must also be rooted in reality.

PRACTICE

Mountain Pose
(Tadasana)

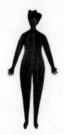

Mountain Pose, the foundation for all standing poses, increases bodily awareness to improve overall posture. The thighs, knees (Capricorn's domain), and ankles are strengthened as the hamstrings release. The abdomen is subtly firmed and the glutes become engaged to support the health and integrity of the lumbar spine, which can relax into the posture.

Like all poses, Tadasana is subjective to an individual body's needs. There is no one way to teach Tadasana, and the shape invites you to explore your own body in space in a way that feels intuitively natural and anatomically wise to you. That might mean anything from changing the positioning of your feet by bringing them closer together or wider apart and slightly turned out, to exploring the center of gravity in your midsection by drawing awareness to your pelvis.

By rooting into the soles of the feet and extending through the crown of the head, clarity is cultivated in the third-eye (ajna) chakra. Grounding into the feet provides the foundation to bring the root (muladhara) chakra into balance.

THIS WEEK: ALIGN WITH YOUR CORE VALUES

Identifying core values allows you to align with dreams, goals, and ideals, and solidify the intentions you wish to set. When we live in accordance with core values, our external actions and behaviors are congruent with our sankalpa. This leads to feelings of contentment, satisfaction, and happiness. When our behavior is misaligned with our values, we may feel lethargic and lacking in purpose, frustrated and depressed, or even angry.

Choose a moment when have you felt happy, fulfilled, and proud. Consider what it was about this situation that made you feel this way, and write it down. Next, recall a time when you felt a sense of regret; write about why this instance made you feel this way. Notice the difference between the two. Set a couple new year's intentions to invite more of the former into your life, so that you may become more of who you wish to be, bolstering more of the person you are already becoming.

DHARMA TALK

An intention is creativity in action
fulfilling our needs for
career or relationships,
money or material things.
An intention must be planted,
like a seed, nourished and
tended to.
But an intention cannot grow
if you do not let it go.
It must be released outwardly
to make itself known.

41

COMMITMENT

Persistence over Resistance

The nature of the mind is chaotic and restless. Buddhists call this the "monkey mind," which prefers to ruminate and fixate as it creates and cycles through complicated stories, whether true or not, on repeat. To cling to these narratives is to give in to fear that is deeply rooted in the ego and resistant to change. When we recognize our patterns, we learn how to overcome them.

Committing to oneself through yoga and meditation is the discipline of displacing those anxieties, to break free from the mind's chatter, and to settle the monkey mind. As we sit, move, and breathe, we quietly consider the realities swirling within and around us, and realize a presence that allows us to navigate our fears from a place of ease and stability.

Patanjali discusses the idea of commitment in sutras 1.20 and 1.21. These lay the groundwork for the second chapter of the *Yoga Sutras,* about the practice in action. Sutra 1.20 states that sraddha (faith), virya (vigor or strength of will), and smrti (memory) are all essential for personal development. We must have faith that we are on the right path, be committed to moving forward, and be willing to learn from our mistakes. Sutra 1.21 suggests that the more keenly intent a practitioner is, the more committed they are to the practice, the more quickly they will move toward understanding their truest nature.

Commitment to this type of work requires truthfulness and authenticity. We should feel secure in our abilities and have faith in our choices without the need for external validation. It is a personal promise to persevere—even when we want to give up. When we set intentions we clarify our thoughts so that we may name them with words. When it comes to committing to those intentions, it is our actions that speak volumes.

Commitment is an appropriate theme for the start of a new year, since Capricorn season is the zodiac's most ambitious cycle. A persistent earth sign ruled by Saturn and symbolized by the mythical Sea Goat, Capricorn can be stoic, stern, and even stubborn. Yet Capricorn also possesses a knack for rooting the loftiest of dreams into tangible reality, committed to seeing a goal through to its completion.

PRACTICE

Plank Pose
(Kumbhakasana)

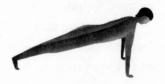

You'd be hard-pressed to find a yogi who doesn't have a love-hate relationship with Plank Pose. With a few basic biomechanical adjustments, this total-body strengthening exercise is more sustainable than we may realize. By placing the hands a bit wider, rather than beneath the shoulders, and pushing the floor away to keep the back body lifted, the pelvis can float in line with the low ribs. As the spine stays neutral (naturally curvy, not flat), Plank also engages the chest and pectoral muscles as the wrist and ankle joints are strengthened. Commit to practicing Plank for up to a minute, lowering to hands and knees whenever rest is needed.

As the abdominal wall fires, the solar plexus (manipura) chakra is activated, fueling the posture with purpose. This illuminates the true self—which, as Picasso said, is all we have: "The sun is a thousand rays in your belly. All the rest is nothing."

THIS WEEK: NAME YOUR EXCUSES

The art of commitment is a path of persistence and focus. It is to align with intention by putting our goals into action, transforming prospect into reality. But first, we must identify our blocks, which we avert or dodge, avoid or run away from, sidestep or deflect. Think of three to five instances when you were presented with an opportunity to make a change, either one you took upon yourself or one that was presented to you, such as a new job or other life-altering endeavor. How did you respond in each instance?

If you're navigating a recent intention, what is your typical internal dialogue? What are the fears that come up that prevent you from fully committing to making that change last? What are your reasons for quitting? Be honest. Whether it's general laziness, lack of time, or financial resources, identify your excuses—your blocks—and write them down. When you're finished, notice any recurring excuses you make and contemplate the root of your fear-based mentality. Can you commit to changing that mentality?

DHARMA TALK

To boldly commit and
embrace with grace
the evolving self
requires not only courage
but practice.
In stillness we stoke the
fires of resilience,
reclaiming the narrative and
recommitting to growth.

BUILDING

The Practice of Habitual Ritual

What are you building? Is it an empire or a home? A stronger body or a stable mind? Is it intentional or haphazard? Whatever it is you are developing, consciously or not, you are creating a practice. A practice is a habit, pattern, or tendency that gives way to a consistent regular routine. Practices are building blocks that make us more resilient.

Yoga is a process of slow and steady building, be it sequencing of physical postures or fostering inner resiliency. The sutras describe our samskaras as inherited karmic patterns that are reinforced through unconscious repetition, in part due to societal conditioning. As we develop awareness for these cyclical patterns, noticing them as they arise, we undo what is outmoded so that we may eventually break free. In this freedom we are able to develop new, healthier habits and build toward the strongest version of ourselves.

Building is a process of determination and grit. Building any-thing—relationships, spaces, businesses, inner knowing—is hard work. Whether you're practicing challenging postures or prolonged pranayama, it takes patience, surrender, and strength. We train our bodies and our minds by building from the ground up. Each time we come to the mat, we are reminded that persistence matters, and we learn to celebrate the small victories.

Just as any building project requires a blueprint, habit building asks us to calculate a practical road map that leads us to where we're going. The French writer, poet, and aviator Antoine de Saint-Exupery said, "A goal without a plan is just a wish." We commit to what we are building by plotting a course. Not all plans need to be seismic changes in our lives. Even small decisions and commitments can create a paradigm shift.

Building new structures invokes the Saturnian energy of earth sign Capricorn, the zodiac's workhorse and methodical taskmaster. Capricorn energy is persistent even in the face of challenge and, as a cardinal sign, is eager to begin projects and take initiative. Capricorn rules the joints in the body and asks us to build stable foundations for our goals so that they are grounded in reality.

PRACTICE

Downward-Facing Dog
(Adho Mukha Svanasana)

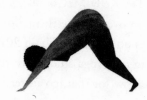

Downward-Facing Dog is one of the most universally known postures and a building block for most other shapes. It's a place of active rest that we revisit throughout practice. Downward Dog is an opportunity to explore your samskaras by allowing the shape to be malleable and adaptable in the moment, rather than rigid or stagnant. What does it feel like to pedal out the feet? Bend and straighten the legs? Take a wider stance?

Benefit from your own personal exploration of the shape by prioritizing neutrality in your spine as you anchor into your palms and feet. Bending the knees allows the spine to neutralize from tailbone to crown. It is not necessary to lower your heels to the floor, nor is it a requirement to straighten your legs. Press the floor away to engage and strengthen the shoulders and arms.

Lengthening the back body in Downward Dog allows prana to travel up and down the spinal cord (sushumna) freely and unblock the chakras. Grounding into the earth through hands and feet engages the root (muladhara) chakra—the foundational opening from which we can begin to build.

THIS WEEK: STRUCTURING NEW ROUTINES

Imagine it is one year from today: What intention or resolution would you most have wanted to stick to? A *New York Times* article provides a few simple science-backed tips for how to stick to new habits, including some from Dr. Kelly McGonigal, who says that it's more productive to choose an overarching theme for the year rather than trying to force routines on ourselves (Shain 2019). So if your resolution is "Go to the gym or a yoga studio five times a week" but the reality of life doesn't allow for that, go instead with a broad theme such as "Make daily movement a priority." A more attainable commitment like this is a small step to reaching a larger milestone.

A steady approach to habit building will feel less routine and more like a way of life. Determine your theme and work backward from there, identifying attainable changes you can make to create healthy new habits that resonate with your resolution.

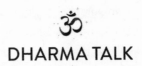

DHARMA TALK

There's nothing mundane
about healthy routines
when we're building new habits
and patterns and dreams.
The ritual of routine
is a process of reframing,
undoing and redoing
unbecoming and becoming
again and again.

AMBITION

Determined Persistence
in Any Pursuit

A memorable line from Shakespeare's *Julius Caesar* is uttered by the title character when he looks to the group of his assailants and sees his friend and ally, Brutus. The words Caesar uttered with his dying breath, "Et tu, Brute?," have become literary shorthand for betrayal—and Brutus an archetype for the ambitious, choosing treachery over loyalty for personal advancement.

Ambition that drives professional gain is necessary and healthy. There is no shame in the pursuit of a fulfilled or comfortable life when aligned with the integrity of our beliefs and morals. But Brutus-like, egocentric ambition blinds us to harm we may cause others, breaking the practice of ahimsa, the yama that instructs non-harming.

In Hindu mythology, the supreme deity is a trinity, representing creation, preservation, and transformation. Lakshmi is the goddess of fortune, material possession, and prosperity, but her fiercest power comes from being a part of the tridevi alongside Saraswati and Parvati. Omnipotence of the supreme deity requires all three goddesses. While Lakshmi's drive leads to accomplishment, it is with

Saraswati's wisdom and Parvati's love that we may pursue ambition intentionally.

At times, ambition on the mat shows up as jealousy or envy of another person's ability or body. When the practice is met with intention to navigate postures from a place of inquiry, ambition teaches perseverance and confidence. When we release ourselves from the confines of comparison, we can safely and clearly work toward our ambitions.

Ambition falls within Capricorn's domain, a masculine, paternal sign opposite the zodiac from maternalistic Cancer. Capricorn is an earth sign, secure in tradition, and works hard to enjoy the fruits of its labor. A cardinal sign, Capricorn is the doer of the zodiac and a highly motivated seeker in any endeavor. Symbolized by the tenacious and proactive Sea Goat, Capricorn's structured productivity is driven by achievement and drive.

PRACTICE

Handstand
(Adho Mukha Vrksasana)

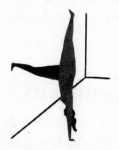

Handstand is an advanced pose of strength and balance, synonymous with ambition. You can learn Handstand at a wall from a shorter Downward-Facing Dog (see page 214). Your palms are the foundation for your base; plug into the heel of the palm, the index fingers, thumbs, and pinky mounds for stability. In this inversion, wrists become ankles and arms become legs.

Lift one leg high and extend through the ball of your foot as though it were an antenna. Come to the ball mound of your grounded foot by lifting your heel, then take a few hops off of that foot. Push into the floor to engage your forearms and triceps, and to allow for shoulder extension. Gaze between your thumbs to extend your cervical spine. Strength in the midback muscles helps protect the lumbar spine from hyperextension—a so-called "banana back." Engagement of the stomach muscles, glutes, and hip flexors helps keep your legs lifted.

As with any inversion, Handstand places your heart above your head, reversing the flow of energy and creating space for new perspectives. Handstand activates the throat (vishuddha) chakra, stimulating the thyroid and regulating metabolism, while externally rotating the shoulders creates space in the heart (anahata) center. As energy flows downward, the crown (sahasrara) chakra is activated.

THIS WEEK: MAKE DREAMS A REALITY

The idea that we have the power to speak things into existence isn't new. Dr. Martin Luther King Jr., in his seminal "I Have a Dream" speech, dared to speak into reality the goals and ambitions of an entire group of people. It's apropos that his birthday falls during Capricorn season. His work is a shining example of how goals can be sought—and achieved, however imperfectly—even in the face of all odds.

As with most things, acknowledging and naming your ambitions is the first step to making them reality. Each morning, determine what it is you desire and speak it into the world. Repeat it to your mirror throughout the day, and say it with conviction.

This doesn't have to be a private exercise. We tend to hold our dreams close to our chest, fearing that we may be judged if we change our minds or because we're embarrassed to fail. While there are certainly some things best kept private, letting loved ones know your ambitions can help keep you accountable on your journey.

DHARMA TALK

There is joy in ambition that speaks
to passion and pursuit—but
be wary of trappings of the ego.
Scarcity is an illusion.
There is room enough for all of us.
So honor your ambition and
celebrate your growth
alongside those beside you.
We are the light each other needs.

INNOVATION

Expanding Boundaries
with New Ideas

There is much debate about certain styles of yoga that speak to the modern age. There's nude yoga, yoga raves, cannabis yoga, yoga with animals, yoga with beer or wine, even death metal yoga. When we picture the great masters—in sepia tones and diaperlike shorts—the advent of some of today's practices may seem jarring, even profane. Yet innovation has long been a crucial part of adapting this practice to an ever-changing world.

B. K. S. Iyengar, considered a contemporary master, was a pioneer of innovation. His introduction of props, for example, was met with resistance in some lineages; many Ashtanga studios still refuse the use of props. For Iyengar, the use of props allowed the mind to find deeper stillness because the body was not stressed but supported—a quality described by Patanjali in sutra 1.33 as "citta prasadanam," serene ordinary consciousness, even in the face of perturbation (Satchidananda 2012).

Innovation in practice can also mean the reconsideration of long-held truths. There are only fifteen poses described in the fifteenth-century *Hatha Yoga Pradipika* (Mohan 2017), while Iyengar's seminal

Light on Yoga (1966) includes more than two hundred. The Ashtanga tradition was developed by Tirumalai Krishnamacharya for young boys as a way for them to expel excess energy. Indra Devi, nee Eugenie Peterson in Russia, was the first woman allowed to be taught by Krishnamacharya. She opened her own school in China and then the United States. Indra's style was significantly different than what Krishnamacharya taught. Tao Porchon-Lynch, the world's oldest yoga teacher at one hundred years old, practiced yoga with young boys in India where she grew up, despite that it was forbidden for girls to participate.

We will never come to know what we don't know without channeling the spirit of invention, by challenging our beliefs and being open to perspectives outside of our own. The postures and sequences we explore are vehicles for expanding our boundaries and adapting accordingly.

As we continue to integrate ancient teachings into modern life, being innovative with our practice is what makes yoga accessible to other communities. But intention matters. Innovations must still ladder to the main objective of yoga, which is to release the mind from the influence of external circumstances, a state Patanjali called pratyahara, the fifth limb of yoga. Otherwise, it's just exercise. Iyengar (1966, 57) writes that the "practice of asanas without the backing of yama and niyama is mere acrobatics."

Innovation is an Aquarian ideal, making Aquarius the inventive trendsetter of the zodiac. An air sign symbolized by the Water Bearer, Aquarius has an energy that is fluid and characterized by deep thinking and high intelligence. This often manifests as tendencies toward science or invention. Aquarius is a fixed sign, meaning that characteristics of depth and determination in evolution can be stubborn or single-minded—somewhat ironic given Aquarian proclivities to change and to resist orthodoxy. Aquarians love problem-solving and can typically be relied on to find an innovative and creative solution.

PRACTICE

Wrist Flip
(Tabletop Variation)

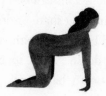

As the world evolves, so does practice to meet modern needs. One example is to stretch the wrists and forearms, ideal given our sustained position on a keyboard or laptop. As innovative Aquarius rules technology, a wrist stretch helps release overtaxed muscles and ligaments from the demands of the digital world.

From a tabletop position, turn your hands out wide (right hand clockwise, left hand counter-clockwise). If this feels okay, try rotating your wrists until your fingertips point toward your knees. According to Katonah Yoga theory, which draws its philosophy from traditional Chinese medicine, stretching the wrists opens and strengthens the lungs (Brower 2017). This allows for increased airflow and longer exhales, activating the parasympathetic nervous system and calming the mind and body.

A broadening of the collarbone allows for an opening of the throat (vishuddha) chakra as the cervical spine (neck) extends. For innovation to last, we need to feel comfortable sharing new ideas, thoughts, or processes. Just as yoga is ever evolving, we too continue to innovate when we collaborate.

THIS WEEK: INVENT YOUR OWN

This book offers weekly rituals to help you home in on your most creative, grounded, and yogic self. What has worked? What hasn't? Evaluate what has resonated and design your own weekly practice that incorporates the best of it. This can be a physical exercise, a journaling exercise, or something you share or do with others. Choose a time of day to repeat—and be flexible with yourself. If you come up with something that just doesn't seem to be working, change it. Developing a weekly practice is hard work. Trust the process and keep challenging your own boundaries and beliefs.

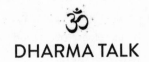

DHARMA TALK

Life does not move forward
without a nudge to do so;
evolution does not come from
maintaining the status quo.
We grow by exploring uncharted maps,
by trusting invention
and seeking the unknown.

COLLABORATION

Freedom Through Interdependence

The hologenome theory is a natural selection process that emphasizes cooperation over competition, which challenges Darwinism and survival of the fittest. It describes the holobiont, an organism that lives together in symbiosis with its bacterial communities and adapts to its surrounding environment. This includes microbial communities: from the vast human microbiome living in the gut and on the skin that work together to keep the immune system in balance, to the larger biomes that exist throughout the diverse ecosystems of our planet.

Michael Pollan (2002) may have alluded to this concept in *The Botany of Desire* when he wrote about coevolutionary relationships. Nature does not exist in a vacuum and neither do we. On a cellular level, everything is interconnected and interdependent, coevolving.

The philosopher Alan Watts (1972) discussed interdependence by connecting it to the Buddhist principle "form is void," meaning that all forms, structures, and organisms are not separate from their backgrounds but connected. Watts describes Earth as a geological entity that grows humans: our existence on this planet is a byproduct of the perfect balance of our solar system, which exists because of the balance in our galaxy, and so on. We are not separate from the divine order of things, nor are we just a cog in the wheel. We are physical manifestations of cosmic creation, cut from the same cloth that weaves together the fabric of the universe.

Collaboration is an Aquarian theme, the sign of group activity and teamwork. During Aquarius season we are encouraged to join forces with others. Aquarius is an innovative air sign ruled by Uranus, a radically minded planet that spins on its side as though it were a celestial act of rebellion, representing high-minded pursuits like spirituality, astrology, and the collective consciousness.

PRACTICE

Triangle Pose
(Trikonasana)

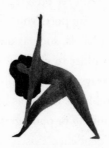

Triangle Pose is a shape of muscular co-contraction. As the psoas and quadriceps of your front leg are activated, you'll find stability in the corresponding hip joint and a deep connection from your back leg to your lumbar. It's common to hyperextend the knees, which is problematic for the joints. Bend your front knee and rest your forearm on your front thigh, or just in front of the inner thigh, for more support as these muscles learn to fire. Your back hand can be placed on your hip to emphasize neutrality in your spine.

This sense of length can help stimulate your throat (vishuddha) and crown (sahasrara) chakras. As your thoracic spine is mobilized, the chest opens, unblocking the heart (anahata) chakra.

THIS WEEK: CONNECT THE DOTS

Mother Teresa said, "I can do things you cannot, you can do things I cannot; together we can do great things." This very book is a collaboration: the authors, friends and colleagues, utilized their different backgrounds and skills to create a unified whole. This exercise is meant to identify the potential collaborations that might exist in your life and discover how to mine them.

Make a list of ten people. They can be coworkers or loved ones or even familiar faces you might see on a regular basis. Next, list one to two ways that each person supports you. Think about their *qualities* rather than their roles or labels, such as describing them as "creative sounding board" or "shoulder to cry on" versus "friend" or "sister." Next, name one to two ways that you support each person with your skills and talents. It could be as simple as being a good listener or the sharing of a craft like cooking or photography.

Note where interdependence exists. Reach out to someone on your list about collaborating in some capacity, if only just for fun. The next time you are feeling lonely or isolated, know that you can lean on some of these connections because you would do the same for them. We're all in this together.

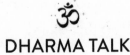

DHARMA TALK

Coming together and staying together,
aligning on a shared vision
and recognizing a single thread—
this is the source of our commonality.
Our humanity reminds us
that we are capable of so much more
when we are not fractured but whole,
when we accept our place in the cosmos.

ELEVATE

Raising Your Vibration

The nature of consciousness and the origin of the soul are two of the greatest mysteries of humankind. Descartes defined consciousness as a spiritual entity devoid of physical law. Others theorize that consciousness is ever-expanding (Goldhill 2016; Koch 2018). Recent advancements in neuroscience begin to explain what Carl Sagan may have alluded to when he described science as a profound source of spirituality (Boyle 2006). The Integrated Information Theory postulates that consciousness can be measured by the brain's capacity for generating neural pathways and processing sensory information (Tononi 2015). This is calculated by phi (ϕ). The more phi measured in the nervous system of an organism, from the smallest insect to a house cat to a human being, the more consciousness it has.

In theoretical physics, consciousness is explored through the lens of quantum nonlocality, which contradicts Einstein's theory of local reality and the laws of classical mechanics. Similar to the idea of non-separability, nonlocality suggests that two particles can continue to interact with each other even when traveling a great distance apart, faster than the speed of light (Goswami 2016). The Dutch author and researcher of near-death studies Pim van Lommel (2011) said, "The mind seems to contain everything at once in a timeless and placeless interconnectedness."

While hard science attests that consciousness begins at the brainstem and dies with the brain (Burkle, Sharp, and Wijdicks 2014), other research explores the possibility of an afterlife (van Lommel 2011, Long 2011). Advocates for transcendental meditation have drawn a parallel between this long-held ideal and that of an eternal, unified consciousness (TMhome.com 2013, Lynch 2007). Some theorists even dub consciousness a new state of matter (Eck 2014). If consciousness is nonlocated, meaning it is neither physical nor separate, could it better be categorized as dark matter? If all matter is made of particles and matter is energy, perhaps consciousness could also be defined as a form of energy.

We have experienced presence and heightened awareness within a yoga or meditation practice, and have witnessed our own expansion of consciousness. We recognize that this expansion is continuous; we understand that the more we know, the less we know. We have all felt an energetic camaraderie among practitioners in group settings, and know on some intrinsic, mysterious level that we are all experiencing something powerfully divine together. As we personally evolve, we elevate each other.

Elevating consciousness is an Aquarian ideal, part of the high-minded sign of the zodiac often described as ahead of its time. Ruled by Uranus, the radical, future-forward-thinking planet, Aquarius reminds us of the power of tapping into the collective conscious and our interdependence with each other and the universe around us.

PRACTICE

Side Plank
(Vasisthasana)

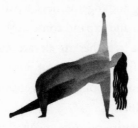

This shape strengthens the abdominal wall and tones the arms and wrists. As the shoulders are stabilized, leg and glute muscles fire. Anchor into the outer edge of your grounded, extended foot to find more balance in the posture. Watch for a tendency to drop the hips, the center of your gravity, and keep your pelvis elevated by engaging your obliques. You can modify Side Plank by stepping your top foot in front of you about halfway up your mat and bending your knee to 90 degrees.

With so much core work happening in this pose, the fires of the solar plexus (manipura) chakra are activated. As the top of the head extends, the crown (sahasrara) chakra is allowed to open to higher insight.

THIS WEEK: ORGANIZE A GROUP MEDITATION

Connecting with like-minded individuals in the physical—and even virtual—"hive mind" has become a great source of inspiration and has fostered belonging and togetherness. Meditation can help us raise our personal vibration and expand consciousness. When we meditate in a group, we come together to elevate consciousness for all of humanity to help shift the structure of our society. When we meditate for peace, love, and happiness, we generate more optimism and elevate our shared reality.

The rise in popularity of large meditation groups like The Big Quiet have shown us that there is something quite profound about this idea. Some mass meditations around the world have even shown a direct impact on lowering crime rate and violence (Chopra n.d.). Organize a group of friends—it doesn't matter how large or small—and put a date on the calendar to meditate together. Afterward, you can listen to your favorite music, spend some quality time over food and drinks, and discuss your experiences.

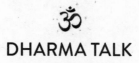

DHARMA TALK

Awareness
is everywhere,
ever present
in all living beings.
To raise our vibration
is a revelation,
an anticipation
of our own elevation—
never separate but together
expanding, cocreating, rising.

REVOLUTION

The Humanitarian Ethos
of Interconnectedness

It is impossible to embody the philosophical tenets of yoga without consideration of our shared social landscape. The philosophical imperative to challenge societal injustice comes from the instruction of ahimsa, the yama of non-harming, and satya, the yama that teaches us to speak our truth. The *Hatha Yoga Pradipika* dictates in chapter 1, verse 15, that "adhering to societal rules" is one of the six causes that destroys the union of yoga. As yogis, we are called to challenge the status quo and revolutionize the rules as we seek this union.

In the 1960s, psychologist Marshall Rosenberg pioneered a form of collaborative conflict resolution known as nonviolent communication (NVC), used in Israel and Palestine, Rwanda, Serbia, Croatia, and South Africa, among others. NVC emphasizes mutual understanding. Because we are all interconnected, the best way to create peace is to get at underlying issues by practicing empathy and compassion, rather than simply "agreeing to disagree."

This requires us to listen as much as to vocalize. This doesn't mean that you must change your beliefs to align with those of another. Revolution is in expanding your consciousness to accept new ideas and beliefs, to adapt what resonates but hold true to your own personal values. It requires tolerance, radical acceptance, and a willingness to work toward necessary change.

Revolution is an Aquarian theme, a social sign fueled by progress and change. Airy Aquarian energy invites fresh perspectives with a humanitarian bent and understands the inner workings of the human condition. This often manifests as idealism to change what is perceived as injustice or maltreatment. Aquarius season is a prime time to act on loftier goals or ambitions spurred by preceding Capricorn. It is when we home in on the interconnectedness of the human experience that revolution is possible.

PRACTICE

Wheel Pose
(Chakrasana or Urdhva Dhanurasana)

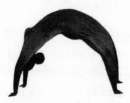

Wheel Pose, also known as Upward-Facing Bow Pose, is an energetic heart opener and backbend that engenders positivity and feelings of goodwill. Its name comes from the same root as "chakra" ("spinning wheel").

Just as chakra theory posits that spinning wheels of energy in our body allow for the flow of energy from root to crown, Wheel represents the completion of a circuit. Beginning on your back provides a connection to the ground from which to rise. Lifting the pelvis and pressing into the hands and feet shifts the weight of the hips above the lower body, initiating a stretch in the lumbar while alleviating work for the arms. Activate your outer hips to avoid compression in the low back. If your hips and shoulders are tight, place blocks under your hands, firm against a wall, and lift to your crown, without placing weight on your head. Alternatively, you may also practice Bridge Pose, beginning supine with a relaxed and neutral spine, and with your knees bent and feet placed outer-hips-width on the floor. Press into the feet to gently lift your hips—without tucking your tailbone under. Arms can be by your sides, or palms interlaced and anchored to the ground.

An energizing pose, Wheel engages all seven chakras. Stimulation of the pituitary and thyroid glands activates the crown (sahasrara) and throat (vishuddha) chakras. The chest lifts, opening the heart (anahata) chakra, giving a boost to feelings of happiness or joy. The backbend opens the back of the solar plexus (manipura) chakra; hugging in the hips to the midline stimulates the sacral (svadhisthana) chakra. Pressing the feet into the ground or blocks activates the root (muladhara) chakra.

THIS WEEK: RADICAL LISTENING

One of the most difficult aspects of humanitarian quest is to put yourself in the shoes of another. Revolution requires empathy and the relegation of our own perception, and it demands that we listen as well as speak. Choosing to actively listen is particularly important when engaging in activism—and it's true for both sides of any debate. Active listening is more than hearing, and it's both surprisingly difficult and rare.

Solicit the help of a trusted friend. Make a list of five questions, beginning with the more superficial ("What's something you're grateful for that happened in the past twenty-four hours?") and gradually becoming more probing ("What frightens you most about death?"). Sit across from each other and set a timer for three minutes. Let one person answer the question without speaking back. Maintain eye contact, and when your mind wanders, bring attention back to your friend. Notice when it becomes difficult and how this may manifest in your daily life. Radical listening is a skill that needs to be practiced—just like asana.

DHARMA TALK

I am you and you are me;
we are not as separate as
it may seem.
It is our greatest joy to
bring light to this union, to
illuminate the shared brilliance
of our interconnected peace.
When we trust in the promise
of true revolution
we find freedom in our
common ground.

CREATIVITY

Quiet Moments of Genius

Ingenuity and imagination are defining characteristics of the human experience. It is our innovation that has—often unconscionably— enabled us to dominate the planet, and it is our creativity that fuels our advancement. Creativity manifests as great works of art, invention, or discovery, but we are all creators. We simply need to give ourselves time and permission to create.

If necessity is the mother of invention, boredom is the mother of creativity. Studies purport that our brains are most creative when they're left to their own devices (instead of being plugged into them). When we daydream, we give our brains permission to explore new patterns of thinking and problem solving (Park, Lim, and Oh 2019).

Absence of sensory stimulation is described in Patanjali's fifth limb of yoga, pratyahara. Pratyahara is the bridge between the external limbs of yoga (yama, niyama, asana, pranayama) and the inner ones (dharana, dhyana, and samadhi). When we quiet the demands of the external world, we are able to tap into the potential of original thought and elevate our unique contributions.

Creativity, however, isn't a solitary pursuit. The theory of multiple discovery, or simultaneous invention, suggests that the bulk of scientific discovery isn't attributable to one particular person but occurs concurrently around the world. One example is the controversy over whether Sir Isaac Newton or Gottfried Wilhelm von Leibniz is the father of calculus; another is the simultaneous invention of the television by five people during the 1920s.

In Hindu lore, Adishakti is the creative energy of the supreme goddess whose third eye, center of intuition and insight, gave birth to Mahasaraswati. Goddess of creativity and consciousness, Saraswati is depicted as having four arms and holding a book, an instrument, and prayer beads.

A creative sign of the zodiac, Pisces is a water sign symbolized by the Fish. Piscean energy was traditionally ruled by Jupiter, the planet of expansion, and is now contemporarily ruled by Neptune, the planet of dreams and creativity. Pisces season is a good time to hunker down with thoughts or in meditation and listen to the meanderings of the mind. It is then that powerful creative impulses can begin to take shape.

PRACTICE

Fish Pose
(Matsyasana)

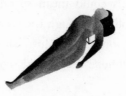

Fish Pose is named for Matsya, the incarnation of Vishnu who saved the future of mankind when he carried the great sages on his back through a devastating flood. Half god, half fish, Matsya was the equilibrium of earth and sea. In order to be creative, we must be stable enough to not be distracted by need and free enough to let our mind wander.

Fish Pose stretches the neck and chest. Press the forearms, just below the ribcage, into the ground to safely extend the spine as the chest lifts. This supported backbend creates space in the ribcage and provides a stretch of the psoas (the muscles connecting the spine to the legs). Rest the back or top of your head on the ground without allowing the breath to constrict. Fish Pose can be made more accessible by placing one block beneath your shoulder blades and another beneath your head. Let your arms relax on either side.

Fish Pose stimulates the creative waters of our sacral (svadhisthana) chakra and helps balance the heart (anahata) chakra. Opening along the throat (vishuddha) chakra allows us to find expression of our creativity, to actualize what we are able to conceive when we create the space to do so.

THIS WEEK: MEDIA DETOX

In our twenty-four-hour news cycle, it can seem imperative to remain fixated on current events. For one week, give yourself a break from certain stimuli in your life that may be inhibiting your imagination's ability to flourish. This could mean spending your mornings in silence rather than scrolling through the morning news, or resisting the temptation to turn on the TV for "background noise." Create parameters around cellphone usage by designating certain hours as phone-free.

Pay close attention to the moments when you feel compelled to fill the void with noise or stimulation. Is being alone with your thoughts uncomfortable? Take note of those feelings—and then watch how your mind begins to replace them. Keep a notebook nearby and write down the random things that float to the surface: an exploration of formerly held beliefs, a memory you haven't remembered in ages, or a new idea. Take stock of your creative process.

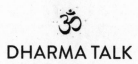

DHARMA TALK

It is in silence
that stories are conceived,
in absence that
creation is possible.
Expression is in the
mind of the beholder.
In the void we find voice,
we listen,
we learn,
we hear.

MYSTICISM

Transcendental Self-Inquiry

Like consciousness, awareness is everywhere. The *Mandukya Upanishad* describes consciousness as having four separate states: waking (jågrat), dreaming (svapna), deep sleep (sushupti), and pure consciousness (turiya). Turiya, a concept utilized by transcendental meditation practitioners, has been described as the superconscious or the ultimate experience of reality and is comparable to the "unified field."

Turiya is transcendence from the worlds of waking (visible body) and dreaming (subtle body)—and even deep, restful sleep (causal body)—where consciousness exists undistracted by the mind. The causal body is described by the doctrine of the three bodies in Hinduism as the last permeable veil of the soul. The sutras describe the five koshas, or sheaths, that conceal the self like layers of an onion; to experience turiya is to go beyond these layers. The Hindu spiritual teacher and yoga master Swami Sivananda described turiya as returning to a state of infinite bliss, a union or yoking of the self (atman) with god or the divine (Brahma; Sivananda 1958).

Through meditation, be it transcendental or Zen, Vedic or mindfulness, we participate in a lifelong process of uncovering the real self—diving deeper into states of higher consciousness, beyond words and thoughts, to the illumination of universal intelligence. Much like the cosmos, this core wisdom is ever-expanding and infinite. Transcendence is an inward exploration, not a destination; it's a never-ending journey of practice and devotion.

Contemplative inquiry provides higher insight about our life's purpose beyond the limitations of the mind. The Upanishads states that without the true self life could not exist, for the self is within all living beings and transcends all: "The Self is everywhere. Bright is the Self, indivisible, untouched by sin, wise, immanent and transcendent; holding the cosmos together" (Easwaran 2007, 58).

The quietness of the winter season is prime for deep introspection and inner reflection, and mysticism can be considered both an Aquarian and Piscean theme. Ruled by Uranus, the radical side-spinning planet, Aquarius is high-minded; its collaborative synergy is associated with the unified field of interconnectedness. Pisces is mystical and ethereal and, as the twelfth and final sign of the zodiac, possesses psychic abilities and a knowingness of the mysterious nature of reality. Pisces is ruled by Neptune, the god of the seas who governs the subconscious and ethereal realm.

PRACTICE

Hero Pose
(Virasana)

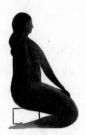

You can sustain Hero Pose for a longer and more comfortable duration by placing a block or two between your ankles (Aquarius's domain) and beneath the base of the coccyx, or tailbone, as the knee joints are stabilized and the quadriceps are stretched. As the Pisces-ruled feet receive a gentle stretch in plantar flexion, your spine can be held upright from the support of your base.

Draw your attention to your third eye (ajna) and envision the crown of your head (sahasrara) opening to higher consciousness, blossoming like a thousand-petaled lotus. Hero Pose can ground the subtle energetic body to stabilize the root (muladhara) chakra and is an appropriate place for connecting to your inner world.

THIS WEEK: NOBLE SILENCE

Vipassana, translated as "insight," is a 2,500-year-old technique used by the Buddha to cultivate higher awareness. It is a practice of developing clear, unobstructed awareness of the present moment. It is a glimpse of reality as it is, by which you can sit in meditation and concentrate on a focal point to break through mental sheaths or layers, and begin to experience pure bliss awareness. Vipassana meditations have become a popular retreat offering, since you can be free from the usual distractions of life.

In Buddhism, vipassana is practiced through "noble silence." Carve out space in your schedule for silent contemplative inquiry without distraction. You can choose to practice noble silence for an entire day, if possible. If not, can you dedicate half of a day—or even a couple of hours—to silence? Engage in a silent solo activity like going for a long walk or hike, free of distractions (including your smartphone). At first, silence can seem uncomfortable and awkward, but try to embrace it. Acknowledge discomfort as it arises, then journal your reflections.

DHARMA TALK

Dive inward
and seek guidance.
Transcendence
is a journey,
not a destination.
The art of inquiry
is a practice
of knowing our real nature,
of shedding what is untrue
to commune with the universal—
the self that is you.

50

HEALING

Embodying Your Own Recovery

Our bodies carry memories just as our minds do. When we experience trauma, our fight-or-flight response engages, accelerating heart-rate and releasing excess cortisol, the stress hormone. When trauma is repeated, patterns are created in the nervous system, disrupting social behaviors with conditioned responses. Pain, grief, and heartache biologically make us anxious, angry, and depressed.

These responses are largely controlled by the vagus nerve, the longest nerve in your body that, oversimplified, is the bridge between impulse and action. The fight-or-flight response corresponds to a low vagal tone. High vagal tone results in a slowed heartbeat, increased digestive function, and overall body regulation. There are many studies that prove how ancient practices of chanting, conscious breathing, and intentional posture can stimulate vagal tone (Porges 2009).

We have all experienced trauma to some degree. Pain and suffering are relative and personal. But even after major blows that render us unable to function normally, we eventually begin to cognitively reorganize our world into one that holds the loss. In our practice, we slow the breath and release into the body, training ourselves to override the body's need to fight. We teach ourselves to physically heal emotional pain and learn, biologically, to let go.

Depression, anxiety, and addiction are some coping mechanisms that we use to bury the effects of trauma. They evoke our shadow selves: feelings of guilt, shame, fear, and judgment. In a state of physical calm, we are able to step into the light and face our darkness with peace, compassion, and joy.

Pisces is the healer of the zodiac and an ethereal, mystical energy that soothes and calms. Empathetic to the point of fault, Pisces can be elusive; such extreme sensitivity comes with a cost. Pisces is also known for its addictive tendencies. Ruled by Neptune, planet of receptivity and ruler of the spirit realm, Pisces attunes us to what plays beneath the surface, much as practice gives insight to the mind. In order to heal, we must be able to look inward with empathy and actively surrender to a place of compassion.

PRACTICE

Supine Pigeon
(Supta Kapotasana)

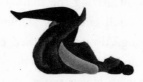

Pigeon is typically practiced folding forward, with one leg bent at the knee and tucked in front of the hips while the other leg extends back. Though ubiquitous in modern vinyasa, this variation can put dangerous asymmetrical pressure on the SI joint—the joint between the pelvis bones.

Supine Pigeon, also known as Supine Figure Four, is more functional and provides the same benefit for an outer hip stretch. Lying on your back takes gravity and body weight off the pelvis. Keep the back of your pelvis anchored to the floor to avoid overexertion in the lower back. Maintain space between your chin and chest as you reach for behind the thigh or the front of your shin to pull the leg toward you. If the pelvis starts to tilt or the shoulders lift, use a strap.

Supine Pigeon activates the sacral (svadhisthana) chakra, our watery seat of emotion and expression. It's often said that we carry our trauma in our hips, though this has not been scientifically proven. But given that the hip is the largest joint in the body, taking measures to keep that joint lubricated is beneficial regardless. Because this pose is supine, it corresponds to the back side of all the chakras. If the front side of our chakras corresponds to conscious reality, the back side represents our connection to the intangible. In order to heal ourselves, we must be able to address the wounds we cannot see.

THIS WEEK: RELEASE WHAT NO LONGER SERVES

When we are in pain, it's our instinct to bury or ignore the source, but in order to move through it, we must first allow it to move through us. This could mean integrating the trauma into everyday life, to temper its power to derail emotional stability. This ritual is not intended to be triggering. Always acknowledge and confront trauma as you are ready to do so, and honor your process.

Call to mind what no longer serves, then gather a handful of items that symbolize whatever it is you're wanting to release. Place these objects in a visible space, then give yourself thirty seconds to ruminate on them each day. Let those thirty seconds become mini meditations—deepen your breathing and surrender to the stillness. Allow your brain to reorganize and reclaim the significance of the objects, turning them into things of beauty and peace. You can, optionally, bury, burn, or otherwise dispose of these objects if and when you're ready.

DHARMA TALK

Life is light but
full, too, of darkness,
and sadness,
and pain.
We have the power to heal,
to move through suffering,
to cultivate strength and perseverance
from a place of beauty and truth.
It is when we acknowledge
the darkness
that we are able to
step into light.

51

ACCEPTANCE

Forgiveness Through Empathy

Carl Jung's collective unconscious theory suggests we are all born with a shared collection of knowledge and imagery inherited from our ancestors. This is different from the collective conscious—belief systems shared by a particular society—and instead refers to an individual's subconscious beliefs and instincts. Jung believed that the human psyche taps into these primal instincts during times of crisis and turmoil (McLeod 2018). If you've ever wondered why you react a certain way when you're triggered or activated by another person or situation, this gives some context as to why.

In sutra 2.3, Patanjali describes the kleshas, our collective obstacles of which we are unaware, as the hindrances we must overcome to understand our real nature. We can look to the kleshas—namely dvesha (aversions) and abhinivesha (fear of death)—to ascertain how certain life events, painful and difficult as they may be, can play an illuminating role in our quest to know ourselves.

When we are caught in dvesha, we are clinging to our pain and carrying it with us, turning to coping mechanisms to manage emotional discomfort. When we forgive ourselves and those who've hurt us, we release ourselves from that pain and transcend from our suffering. Abhinivesha speaks to our personal—and collective—fear of dying. Fear holds us back from knowing ourselves and shrouds reality in false illusion mired in distractions, attachments, ego, and ignorance. When we learn to accept the ways things are, we can more readily let things be. We may even learn to accept that one day we too will die.

Accepting mortality begins with forgiveness; forgiving ourselves first is the hardest part. It means looking deep within our subconscious, into the darkest shadows, and accepting that we are enough. Forgiveness illuminates the recesses of our unconscious mind to reveal patterns and triggers—and teaches us how to coexist with them. Learning to accept trauma as part of our story allows us to forgive ourselves, so that we may forgive others. By recognizing that we are all suffering, we develop empathy even toward those who've hurt us. Through practice and experience, it becomes possible to accept the necessary dark and difficult as much as the light and easy.

Forgiveness manifests during the quiet solitude of the winter season. Ruled by Neptune, the planet of the psyche and subconscious, Pisces season marks the final astrological cycle before we are renewed again come spring. Pisces is the healer and mystic of the zodiac, and known for its psychic abilities. Practicing acceptance is appropriate any time of year, but Pisces season awakens our capacity for empathy.

PRACTICE

Simple Spinal Twist
(Supta Matsyendrasana Variation)

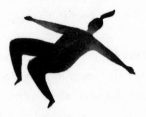

This variation of Reclined Spinal Twist places less torque on the spine. Open your arms to a T or cactus shape, and widen your feet to the edges of your mat, so that you can allow the knees to drop to each side more naturally without tugging on the psoas or the muscles in your lower back. This posture activates the parasympathetic nervous system to calm and relax the body and mind.

As the abdominal muscles and organs are gently stimulated, the sacral (svadhisthana) and solar plexus (manipura) chakras activate. As the spine realigns, all seven chakras from root to crown are roused in this restful shape.

THIS WEEK: AIR YOUR GRIEVANCES

Empathy-motivated forgiveness is the ability to empathize with another person, despite how they have hurt you. Conflicts are inevitable in life and especially in our relationships. When we realize that our transgressors have their own pain, suffering, sadness, shame, and guilt, we can understand that they too are only human.

Make two lists. In the first, name some of your biggest mistakes, wrongdoings, or moments that brought you guilt or regret. Be sure to include anyone you may have hurt as a result of those actions. Next, forgive yourself for each item on your list. Write down each act of forgiveness and/or say it out loud.

The next list is for everyone in your life who has hurt you. Name them, and then one by one acknowledge that each person came into this world with their own karmic inheritances and suffers in their own way. Can you forgive them? Is there anyone you feel compelled to reach out to?

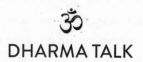

DHARMA TALK

It takes real courage
to forgive ourselves,
to forgive another.
It takes real love
and self-acceptance
to forgive ourselves,
and especially each other.
If compassion
is love in action,
then forgiveness
is acceptance
of our imperfections,
flaws and all.

52

DEATH

The Release

Humans have attempted to explain death with deities and mythologies since before recorded time; religious ideas have shaped sociopolitical context for centuries. Despite scientific advances and a millennia of artistic musing, we are no closer to understanding life's greatest unknown. Regardless, death is one of life's foundational certainties, transcending time, place, and circumstance. The one thing we cannot explain is the one thing that resolutely binds us.

Aparigraha is, fittingly, the last of the yamas described by Patanjali and instructs non-attachment. Accepting the body's mortality is the ultimate practice of aparigraha. We need not believe in the transmigration of souls—or avoid grieving someone we love—to view the physical body through this lens.

The mortal suffering of birth, death, and rebirth is known in Hindu and yogic theory as samsara. Unification with the divine consciousness breaks this cycle. Patanjali writes that practicing the eight limbs of yoga (yama, niyama, asana, pranayama, pratyahara, dharana, dahyana, and samadhi) leads to this unification. This, like all beliefs about what happens in death, is a personal, subjective truth—personal satya. Death is biology's satya. How we approach death is our own.

Yoga is, at its core, the acceptance of our mortality. Yoking body and mind distills the chatter, so that we can arrive fully in the present. Acting with empathy by accepting our interconnectedness creates communities of compassion and kindness. Acceptance of our body's temporality—of death—allows us to keep moving forward, rekindling our will to live and let live.

Death belongs to the realm of Pisces, the last sign of the zodiac, the completion of the astrological year. Pisces is the great empath and dreamer of the zodiac, ruled by Neptune, planet of the spiritual world. Neptune's energy inspires intuition and sensitivity, teaching us to approach that which we cannot explain from a place of integrated truth and compassion.

The winter months culminate with Pisces season, before the astrological calendar resets with Aries season and signifies the birth of a new life cycle.

PRACTICE

Corpse Pose
(Savasana)

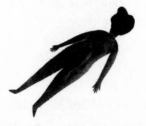

Though it appears deceptively easy, Corpse Pose is arguably one of the most difficult asanas. Commonly offered at the end of practice, Savasana is the full integration of body and mind—awareness of, but not control over, the breath—and asks us to sink into the absolute present, releasing any manipulation of body. It is complete and utter surrender.

Spending time in constructive rest, with your knees bent and soles of your feet on the floor, before entering Savasana can help reset your nervous system. Lying on your back with your feet on the ground a few inches from your seat allows your psoas muscles to release. Shortened, tight psoas muscles can restrict our ability to breathe deeply, making us anxious. Constructive rest also helps to alleviate tension in the low back and pelvis.

Extend your legs and arms in a way that feels comfortable, allowing your body to surrender to gravity. If there is any tension in your lower back or neck, place a rolled-up blanket or bolster beneath your knees or neck, respectively. Asymmetry is natural—there is no need to lie with limbs perfectly arranged around the body. Savasana enhances proprioception, a chance to notice and honor our asymmetries.

Savasana is a grounding pose, activating the root (muladhara) chakra. It engages the primary curves of the spine, the sacral and thoracic curvatures, those that form fully in the womb. This stimulates the sacral (svadhisthana) chakra, seat of primordial creativity and passion, and the heart (anahata) chakra, seat of acceptance and intrinsic wholeness.

THIS WEEK: TENSE-AND-RELEASE BODY SCAN MEDITATION

To recognize and accept the temporality of our bodies, we must first acknowledge and release. Lie comfortably in Savasana. Deepen the breath while the mind and body settle, and establish a steady rhythm of inhales and exhales. Then concentrate all your attention on one leg. On an inhale, tense all the muscles in that leg for five seconds. Exhale and release. Repeat on the other leg. Do the same on each arm, and then the core, being mindful of the low back. Finally, scrunch the muscles of the face together, squeezing eyes closed and pursing the lips. Hold and release.

Repeat or remain in Savasana, letting the mind rest without concentration on the breath.

ॐ

DHARMA TALK

Death is beginning as well as end;
from the ash comes new growth,
from each sunrise the dawn.
There is no choice but surrender—
years come, seasons change.
Stars will always have their night
and the fields their sun-kissed dew.
Fear not the great unknown.
It has been with you all along.

Acknowledgments

To our friends, families, companions, colleagues, and collaborators for your support and encouragement of our journey as writers over the years: Finn Cohen, Ryan Cheresson, Hillary Johnson, Alicia Rice, Jim Johnson, Kossi Yawli, Dan Rice, Kathy Rice, Shirley Rice, Maureen Maguire Lewis, Lauren Enos, Elizabeth Kessler, John W. Wright, Elizabeth Christensen, Meghan Conway, Jordan Fleet, Sharon O'Neal, Robert Sturman, Amy and Aaron Goodykoontz, Brian Colgan, Mara Mayer, Kerri Shaw, Megan Robertson, Campbell Ringel, Mary Hodges, Grace Edquist, Amanda Kohr, Kelsey Savage, Mollie Earls, Karina Mackenzie, Steve Berman, Ryan LeMere, Kim Small, Gabbi Archambault, and Molly, Bela, Lenny, and Kali.

And also to those who left us too soon: the late Karen Johnson and Jack Rice.

To our mentors, teachers, and heroes, for your shared collective wisdom that—whether you may know it or not—has inspired and informed this book: Ophira and Tali Edut, Alexandria Crow, Elena Brower, Leslie Kaminoff, Monica Shannon, Linda Sparrowe, Dani Shapiro, Schuyler Grant, Mary Beth LaRue, Dr. Chelsea Jackson Roberts, Chelsey Korus, Eoin Finn, Carmen Curtis, Noah Maze, and Donovan McGrath.

To the studios that have sustained us and the students who've given us the space to share and sharpen our voices: blue lotus yoga & movement arts, Daya Yoga Studio, SHAKTIBARRE, shambhala yoga & dance; especially Jill Sockman, Deborah Ross, Liisa Ogburn,

Sarah Schumann, Rachel Ginsberg, Colin Ilsley, Ali Abate, Jonathan Carl Flemister, Ania Lesniak, Carmina Rodrigues, Corinne Wainer, Debby Siegel, Cameron Tolle, and Alfie Dumlao.

And to our editor, Vicraj Gill, for her dedication and patience, as well as to our acquisitions editor, Ryan Buresh, for believing in this project and giving us the opportunity to bring it into the world.

Our heartfelt gratitude goes out to all of you.

The Astrological Wheel of Life

COSMIC EMBODIMENT

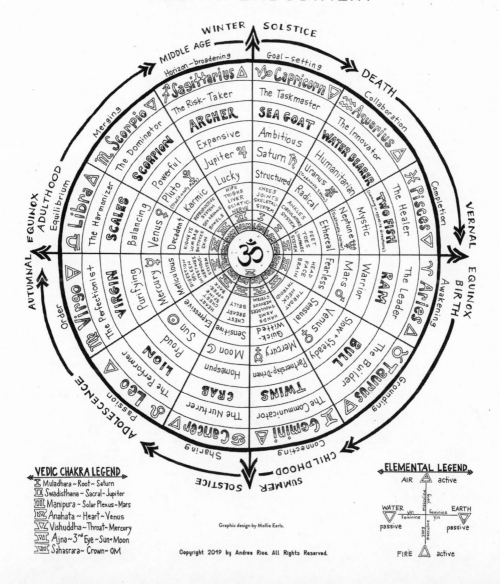

Recommended Reading

Autobiography of a Yogi. P. Yogananda. London, UK: Rider, 1955.

The Bhagavad Gita. Introduced and translated by Eknath Easwaran. Tomales, CA: Nilgiri Press, 2007.

Be Here Now. Ram Dass. San Cristobal, NM: Lama Foundation, 1971.

Big Magic: Creative Living Beyond Fear. Elizabeth Gilbert. New York: Riverhead Books, 2016.

Catching the Big Fish: Meditation, Consciousness, and Creativity. David Lynch. New York: Deckle Edge, TarcherPerigee, a Penguin Group imprint, 2017.

The Complete Mahabharata. Ramesh Menon. Mumbai, India: Repro Knowledgcast Ltd., 2017.

Eastern Body, Western Mind: Psychology and the Chakra System as a Path to the Self. Anodea Judith. Berkeley, CA: Celestial Arts, 2004.

The Hatha Yoga Pradipika: Translation with Notes from Krishnamacharya. Translation by A. G. Mohan. Svastha Yoga, 2017.

Inward. Yung Pueblo. Kansas City, MO: Andrews McMeel Publishing, 2017.

Kamasutra. Vatsyayana. CreateSpace Independent Publishing Platform, 2016.

The Key Poses of Yoga. Ray Long. Austin, TX: Greenleaf Book Group, 2008.

The Life-Changing Magic of Tidying Up: The Japanese Art of Decluttering and Organizing. Marie Kondo. Berkeley, CA: Ten Speed Press, 2014.

Light on Yoga. B. K. S. Iyengar. New York: Allen & Unwin, Knopf Doubleday Publishing Group, 1966.

The Miracle of Mindfulness: An Introduction to the Practice of Meditation. Thich Nhat Hanh. Translated by Mobi Ho. New York: Beacon Press, 1999.

The Natyasastra: English Translation with Critical Notes. Adya Rangacharya. Revised Edition. New Delhi: Munshiram, 2014.

Practice You: A Journal. Elena Brower. Sounds True, 2017.

The Prophet. Kahlil Gibran. New York: Alfred A. Knopf, 1966.

Ramayana. C. Rajagopalachari. Mumbai, India: Bharatiya Vidya Bhava, 1951.

Still Writing: The Perils and Pleasures of a Creative Life. Dani Shapiro. New York: Grove Press, 2014.

The Sun and Her Flowers. Rupi Kaur. Kansas City, MO: Andrews McMeel Publishing, 2017.

Tao Te Ching. Laozi. Translated and with commentary by Roger T. Ames and David L. Hall. New York: Ballantine Books, 2004.

The Upanishads. Introduced and translated by Eknath Easwaran. Tomales, CA: Nilgiri Press, 2007.

Wheels of Life: A User's Guide to the Chakra System. Anodea Judith. Woodbury, MN: Llewellyn Publications, 1987.

When Things Fall Apart: Heart Advice for Difficult Times. Pema Chödrön. Berkeley, CA: Shambhala, 2016.

Yoga Anatomy. Leslie Kaminoff and Amy Matthews. Champaign, IL: Human Kinetics Publishers, 2011.

The Yoga Sutras of Patanjali. Translation and commentary by Sri Swami Satchidananda. Reprint edition. Buckingham, VA: Integral Yoga Publications, 2012.

References

Akandere, M., and B. Demir. 2011. "The Effect of Dance over Depression." *Collegium Antropologicum* 35(3): 651–6.

Beermann, U., and W. Ruch. 2011. "Can People Really Laugh at Themselves? Experimental and Correlational Evidence." *Emotion* 11: 492–501.

Borowski, Susan. 2012. "Quantum Mechanics and the Consciousness Connection." American Association for the Advancement of Science. Accessed November 28, 2018. https://www.aaas.org/quantum-mechanics-and-consciousness-connection.

Boyle, Alan. 2006. "Retracing Carl Sagan's Spiritual Quest." NBCNEWS.com. May 3. Accessed February 6, 2019. http://www.nbcnews.com/id/12615326/ns/#.XNiT5NNKjow.

Brower, Elena. 2017. "A Heart-Opening Yoga Sequence with Elena Brower." *Yoga Journal.* Accessed January 18, 2019. https://www.yogajournal.com/practice/elena-brower-heart-opening-yoga-sequence.

Burkle, C., R. Sharp, and E. Wijdicks. 2014. "Why Brain Death Is Considered Death and Why There Should Be No Confusion." *Neurology* 83(16): 1,464–69. Doi: 10.1212/WNL.0000000000000883.

Chopra, Deepak. N.d. "The Power of Group Meditation." The Chopra Center. Accessed February 6, 2019. https://chopra.com/articles/the-power-of-group-meditation.

Clayton, M., R. Sager, and U. Will. 2004. "In Time with the Music: The Concept of Entrainment and Its Significance for Ethnomusicology." *ESEM CounterPoint* (1). http://www.open.ac.uk/Arts/experience/InTimeWithTheMusic.pdf.

Dalai Lama. 1990. "Universal Responsibility and the Environment," excerpt from *My Tibet* by H.H. the Fourteenth Dalai Lama. London: Thames and Hudson Ltd. Accessed March 1, 2019. https://www.dalailama.com/messages/environment/universal-responsibility.

Easwaran, E. 2007. The Bhagavad Gita. 2nd edition. Introduced and translated by Eknath Easwaren. Tomales, CA: Nilgiri Press.

Easwaran, E. 2007. The Upanishads. 2nd edition. Introduced and translated by Eknath Easwaran. Tomales, CA: Nilgiri Press.

Eck, Allison. 2014. "Physicists Say Consciousness Might Be a State of Matter." *Nova Next*, PBS. April 22. Accessed February 6, 2019. https://www.pbs.org/wgbh/nova/article/physicists-say-consciousness-might-be-a-state-of-matter/.

Einstein, A. N.d. "Is the Universe Friendly?" Awakin.org. Accessed November 28, 2018. http://www.awakin.org/read/view.php?tid=797.

Emmons, Robert. 2010. "Why Gratitude Is Good." *Greater Good Magazine*. University of California, Berkeley. Accessed November 1, 2018. https://greatergood.berkeley.edu/article/item/why_gratitude_is_good.

Gaia staff. N.d. "Viparita Karani: The Legs Up the Wall Pose." *Gaia*. Accessed February 5, 2019. https://www.gaia.com/article/viparita-karani-legs-wall-pose.

Goldhill, Oliva. 2016. "Scientists Say Your Mind Is Confined to Your Brain, or Even Your Body." *Quartz*. December 24. Accessed February 5, 2019. https://qz.com/866352/scientists-say-your-mind-isnt-confined-to-your-brain-or-even-your-body/.

Goswami, A. 2016. "An introduction to Quantum Activism." Amit Goswami.org. March 23. Accessed February 6, 2019. https://www.amitgoswami.org/2016/03/23/an-introduction-to-quantum-activism/.

Iyengar, B. K. S. 1966. *Light on Yoga*. New York: Allen & Unwin, Knopf Doubleday Publishing Group.

John Hopkins Medicine. N.d. "The Power of Positive Thinking." Johns Hopkins University, Baltimore, MD. Accessed December 3, 2018. https://www.hopkinsmedicine.org/health/wellness-and-prevention/the-power-of-positive-thinking.

Keysers, C., and V. Gazzola. 2014. "Hebbian Learning and Predictive Mirror Neurons for Actions, Sensations and Emotions." *Philosophical Transactions of the Royal Society B: Biological Sciences* (369). https://doi.org/10.1098/rstb.2013.0175.

Koch, Christof. 2018. "What Is Consciousness?" *Scientific American*. June 1. Accessed February 5, 2019. https://www.scientificamerican.com/article/what-is-consciousness/.

Laozi. 2004. Dao De Ching. Translated and with commentary by Roger T. Ames and David L. Hall. New York: Ballantine Books.

Lee, C. 2010. "Do Less, Relax More: Legs-Up-the-Wall Pose." *Yoga Journal.* August 25. Accessed February 5, 2019. https://www.yogajournal.com /practice/legs-up-the-wall-pose.

Lennon, J., and Yoko Ono. 1980. "Beautiful Boy (Darling Boy)." Double Fantasy. Geffen.

Lesté, A., and J. Rust. 1984. "Effects of Dance on Anxiety." *Perceptual and Motor Skills* 58(3): 767–772.

Loder, Vanessa. 2014. "The Power of Vision: What Entrepreneurs Can Learn from Olympic Athletes." *Forbes.* Accessed November 28, 2018. https://www.forbes.com/sites/vanessaloder/2014/07/23/the-power-of -vision-what-entrepreneurs-can-learn-from-olympic-athletes/#d9 e23776e749.

Long, J. 2011. *The Science of Near-Death Experiences.* San Francisco: HarperOne.

Lynch, D. 2017. *Catching the Big Fish: Meditation, Consciousness, and Creativity.* New York: Deckle Edge, TarcherPerigee, a Penguin Group imprint.

Maslow, A. H. 1943. "A Theory of Human Motivation." *Psychological Review* 50(4): 370–396.

McLeod, Saul. 2018. "Carl Jung." *Simply Psychology.* Accessed March 5, 2019. https://www.simplypsychology.org/carl-jung.html.

Messerly, J. 2014. "Summary of Sartre's Theory of Human Nature." *Reason and Meaning.* November 20, 2014. Accessed November 21, 2018. https://reasonandmeaning.com/2014/11/20/theories-of-human-nature -chapter-18-sartre-part-1/.

Mohan, A. G. 2017. *The Hatha Yoga Pradipika: Translation with Notes from Krishnamacharya.* Translatd by A.G. Mohan. Svastha Yoga.

Nhat Hanh, Thich. 2008. "The Fertile Soil of Sangha." *Tricycle Magazine.* Accessed March 9, 2019. https://tricycle.org/magazine/fertile-soil -sangha/.

Park, G., B.-C. Lim, and H. S. Oh. 2019. "Why Being Bored Might Not Be a Bad Thing After All." *Academy of Management Discoveries* 5(1).

Pollan, Michael. 2002. *The Botany of Desire.* New York: Random House.

Porges, Stephen. 2009. "The Polyvagal Theory: New Insights into Adaptive Reactions of the Autonomic Nervous System." *Cleveland Clinic Journal of Medicine* 76(Suppl 2): S86–S90.

Satchidananda, Sri Swami. 2012. *The Yoga Sutras of Patanjali*. Reprint edition. Translated with commentary by Sri Swami Satchidananda. Buckingham, VA: Integral Yoga Publications.

Schwartz, Stephan. 2018. "The Role of Nonlocal Consciousness in Creativity and Social Change." *EC Psychology and Psychiatry* 7(10): 665–678.

Shain, Susan. 2018. "How to Crush Your Habits in the New Year with the Help of Science." *The New York Times*. December 31. Accessed January 10, 2019. https://www.nytimes.com/2018/12/31/smarter-living/better-habits-tips-new-year-resolutions-science.html.

Sivananda, Sri Swami. *Philosophy of Dreams*. Tehri-Garhwal, Uttaranchal, Himalayas, India: The Divine Life Society.

Sonnenburg, J., and E. Sonnenburg. 2015. "Gut Feelings: The 'Second Brain' in Our Gastrointestinal Systems." *Scientific American* May 9.

Tononi, G. 2015. "Integrated Information Theory." *Scholarpedia* 10(1): 4, 164. doi:10.4249/scholarpedia.4164.

TMhome.com. 2013. "Unified Fields of Consciousness. ONE = MANY." *Transcendental Meditation*. July 15. Accessed February 6, 2019. https://tmhome.com/news-events/unified-field-of-consciousness-onemany/.

Van Lommel, P. 2011. *Consciousness Beyond Life: The Science of the Near-Death Experience*. San Francisco: HarperOne.

Watts, Alan. 1972. "Nothingness." Filmed in 1972. Episode 1, *The Essential Lectures of Alan Watts* series, 28:00. Accessed March 5, 2019. https://www.gaia.com/video/nothingness.

Williams, F. 2017. *The Nature Fix: Why Nature Makes Us Healthier, Happier, and More Creative*. New York: W. W. Norton & Co.

Williamson, Marianne. 2014. *The Law of Divine Compensation: On Work, Money, and Miracles*. New York: HarperCollins.

Zickl, D. 2017. "5 Things I Learned From Throwing My Legs Up a Wall Every Day." *Runner's World*. April 28. Accessed February 5, 2019. https://www.runnersworld.com/health-injuries/a20866611/5-things-i-learned-from-throwing-my-legs-up-a-wall-every-day/.

Lisette Cheresson is a writer, editorial director, and content consultant specializing in wellness, sustainability, and women's empowerment. She has made short films with leaders such as Eddie Stern, Eoin Finn, and Elena Brower; and is an award-winning journalist whose work has appeared in *The Wanderlust Journal*, *Quilt*, *Matador*, the *New York Times* reference books *Off Track Planet*, and others. She completed her 200-hour yoga training in New York, NY; and her Reiki attunement in India. She also studied with Leslie Kaminoff of The Breathing Project, and attended a three-day intensive discourse with the Dalai Lama. She has offered workshops with Wanderlust Festivals and Manifest Station, and completed her end-of-life doula training in 2019. She lives with her husband and animals in the Hudson Valley in New York.

Andrea Rice is a writer and editor covering health and wellness. Her work has appeared in *Yoga Journal*, *The Wanderlust Journal*, *mindbodygreen*, *Astrostyle*, *SONIMA*, and *New York Yoga+Life*. She has also worked as a journalist for the *New York Times* and *INDY Week*. As a yoga teacher with a decade of experience, Andrea completed her 200-hour training in New York, NY; and furthered her training with Elena Brower and Alexandria Crow. She has also studied astrology extensively with The AstroTwins, Ophira and Tali Edut. Andrea has offered yoga, meditation, journaling, and creativity workshops in Brooklyn and Manhattan in New York, and has been a presenter at Wanderlust Festivals in Vermont. She lives in Raleigh, NC, with her husband and their cat.

MORE BOOKS for the SPIRITUAL SEEKER

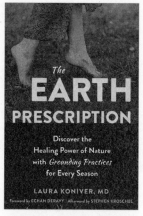

ISBN: 978-1684034895 | US $16.95

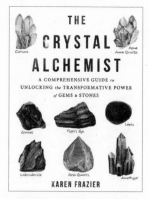

ISBN: 978-1684032952 | US $17.95

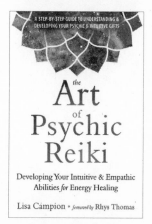

ISBN: 978-1684031214| US $19.95

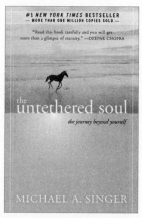

ISBN: 978-1572245372 | US $17.95

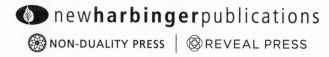